Intermittent fasting for women

The ultimate beginner guide to burn fat, weight loss, learn the healing power of your body through the autophagy and live a healthy lifestyle

[Dr Steven Green]

Upon using the contents and information contained in this book, you agree to hold harmless the Author from and against any damages, costs, and expenses, including any legal fees potentially resulting from the application of any of the information provided by this book. This disclaimer applies to any loss, damages or injury caused by the use and application, whether directly or indirectly, of any advice or information presented, whether for breach of contract, tort, negligence, personal injury, criminal intent, or under any other cause of action.

You agree to accept all risks of using the information presented inside this book.

You agree that by continuing to read this book, where appropriate and/or necessary, you shall consult a professional (including but not limited to your doctor, attorney, or financial advisor or such other advisor as needed) before using any of the suggested remedies, techniques, or information in this book.

Table of Contents

INTRODUCTION

Intermittent fasting has gained popularity in recent years. Hundreds of books and articles have already been written about it. No one can blame these authors since it is a revolutionary way of achieving weight loss. There is no diet. All you have to do is time when you eat and do not eat. Unfortunately, a lot of the information written were created with a male audience or men and women, in general, in mind.

This is where the problem becomes evident. What is written for men rarely applies to women. The body of a man works different to that of a woman and vice versa. Therefore, it is only natural for women to react differently to intermittent fasting. And, as you would find out, this is actually the case.

Moreover, given that there's a difference with how it affects men and women, the methods, tips, and solutions written for men might not actually be effective for women. Women might actually be placing their health at risk by following advice meant for the opposite sex.

It is for this reason that this book was written. This book aims to look at intermittent fasting and see how it can specifically affect women. It looks into the effects and benefits for their health. It would also look into how women can do intermittent fasting in a way that suits them best.

Aside from this, this book would delve deeper into the aspects of intermittent fasting. There a lot of talk about its effects on weight and fat loss. But, it is rarely discussed that intermittent fasting can do so much more than just helping people lose weight. In fact, with its potential benefits for your health, it can be said that everyone should actually do intermittent fasting using one of the methods available.

Intermittent fasting triggers a reaction in your body that is essential to its survival, longevity, and overall health. From a book wherein its audience would probably expect to talk only about fat loss, this book goes so much deeper that it delves into disease prevention, mental enhancement, and potential degenerative disease treatment. Of course, proper research was done to ensure that what is provided in this book can be applied to your life.

Furthermore, this book will provide you with the tools to implement the strategy that will help you have an easier time achieving your goal. It will also clarify some misunderstandings about it and fix some misconceptions about intermittent fasting, weight loss, and diet. It will also provide information on what you need to get started and why you need them.

After reading this book, you will have a better understanding of intermittent fasting, its mechanics, and its actual method. You will also have an idea on how you can do intermittent fasting in a way that works best for your physiology, health condition, preferences, and lifestyle. You will even be given a guide on how to make intermittent fasting easier or, at the very least, more manageable for you. You will also be equipped on how to go about when changing your goals.

From all of these, you will know everything you need to know to get started with intermittent fasting immediately. The only thing missing is for you to start and take action.

Chapter 1: What is Fasting?

At this point, you are probably bursting with questions about what fasting is and how to do it. This chapter answers those questions. You should leave this chapter feeling more knowledgeable and confident in beginning your fasting journey.

Fasting can seem like a daunting task because the media makes it seem extreme (such as extended hunger strikes or weeklong fasts). Fasting simply means you are going without food for a set time period, which could be as little as 12 hours, and is a natural part of our everyday lifestyle and biological metabolic processes. Unfortunately, fasting and severe calorie restriction tend to get paired together even though they are not synonymous.

Fasting is simply a break from food intake—a break that is defined by its duration or intervals, and as part of an otherwise well-balanced eating style that promotes health and energy needs. That is why fasting will not cause any type of serious suffering. Fasting happens naturally for most of us on a daily basis without us even realizing it. Every night while you sleep, you are fasting, unless you happen to wake up for a midnight refrigerator raid. The first meal after you awaken is called "breakfast" for a reason: You are breaking the fast when you consume your morning meal.

THE IMPORTANCE OF HEALTHY FASTING

This book focuses on fasting healthfully and in a way that can help promote and stimulate positive health outcomes. Fasting does this by providing a metabolic reset. Without sounding too buzzwordy, your metabolism can become sluggish over time and require a jump-start to run at full speed again. A sluggish metabolism often limits your potential to reach your health goals. To gain the results desired, such as personal body goals, staying youthful, having efficient digestion, or staying mentally sharp, eating must be approached in a thoughtful, strategic, healthful, and responsible way. I aim to provide you with the information about how fasting can help this process.

I will guide you through popular fasting methods, inform you of how fasting affects a woman's body, the myths surrounding the practice, and the many potential health benefits you may reap from fasting. As you keep reading, learning more, and following the book's advice, it is important you stay true to the guidelines and not attempt to accelerate the process by extending periods of fasting or consuming fewer calories than your body needs. Fasting is, at its core, a way to achieve balance, and balance is not the result of extremes.

SAFETY SIGNALS

Whenever you change your diet, you want to be very aware of how it affects your overall health and be mindful of not risking your safety. Some side effects are bound to occur. Initially experiencing mild to moderate hunger, a little fatigue, and potential moodiness is common as your body adjusts to changes. These symptoms should subside and not seriously affect your health long term. However, your body may reject or resist a new process. If, at any point while fasting, you feel dizzy, faint, nauseated, or experience shaking, migraines, or other indications that you are seriously unwell, it is time to eat. You would be wise to have a nourishing meal and reevaluate what might need adjustment in the future.

MYTHS ABOUT FASTING

When it comes to eating or any popular health topic, real information tends to get obscured by plenty of fake stuff. Let's clarify some of the misconceptions and myths surrounding the topic before moving on to the how-to sections. Here are the most commons questions I've received:

Is fasting unhealthy? Not at all! Short-term fasting is a natural process that most of us experience daily without even noticing.

What is the difference between fasting and intermittent fasting? Technically, all fasting for health reasons is considered intermittent fasting because it is designed to start and stop. This book uses the terms interchangeably.

Isn't not eating food the same as having an eating disorder? No, these are very different things. Eating disorders come from a place of mental control, fear surrounding food choices, and a distorted relationship with how food affects health. Those who fast tend to have a very healthy, positive relationship with food and use the prescribed periods of eating to nourish their bodies thoughtfully.

I've heard that if you don't eat, your body goes into "starvation mode." Is this true? If you eat far less than your body needs for extended periods of time, then yes, your body will work to preserve the stores it has instead of burning them. However, fasting, when done correctly, does not put your body in this compromised position.

Will fasting make my blood sugar drop too low? For most people, fasting works to stabilize and regulate blood sugar levels, allowing your body to have more consistent energy levels.

I want to keep my muscle mass. Will fasting cause my body to eat away at my muscles? Fasting can accelerate fat burning and retain muscle mass. Used in conjunction with a good exercise plan, this process can help you achieve a lean physique.

Won't fasting deprive my body of nutrients? The variety of nourishing foods you'll consume when not fasting is sufficient to sustain your body's needs through fasting periods.

Can't going without food mess up my metabolism? The fact that fasting is intermittent—meaning it starts and stops—helps rev up (not mess up) your metabolism.

If I can't eat, won't I be hangry and cranky? Not eating affects each person's mood differently. If you do experience negative moods, they are likely to pass as your body adjusts to the fast. Also, most of your fast can be done while you're sleeping, if that style works best for you.

I'm worried I'll just binge when I start eating again. Should I be concerned? The process might take a little adjusting to, but fasting should improve and regulate your hunger-satiety levels and cues, allowing your body to eat appropriately for its needs.

I have diabetes. Can I still fast? Fasting can benefit many chronic health conditions by helping to regulate internal factors. If you have a preexisting medical condition, you should consult with a physician before making any lifestyle changes.

I want to keep working out. Isn't that dangerous to do if I'm fasting? You won't have to give up your exercise routine to fast. Fasting workouts can help provide performance adaptations. You'll want to pay attention to your energy levels and adjust the timing of fasting and eating periods to match your workout needs.

Won't fasting mess up my female hormones? When done properly, intermittent fasting can be an effective tool in balancing female hormones. We will touch more on this throughout the book.

THE THREE MAIN METHODS OF FASTING

Now that we've cleared up some common concerns and misconceptions around intermittent fasting, let's dive more into what fasting is. Recall that fasting is the absence of caloric intake for set periods of time. Doing so healthfully requires planning. As a quick introduction to the main styles of fasting for weight loss and health, consider the following:

Time-restricted feeding: In this method, the fasting window spans 10 to 16 hours a day and the remaining hours are non-fasting. During fasting hours, no calories from food or liquid are consumed. Non-caloric substances such as black coffee, water, and plain tea can be enjoyed while fasting. This approach is great for beginners, as a large part of the fasting hours can be spent sleeping and limits the burden of going without fuel. Time-restricted feeding is also known as daily fasting and encompasses the Crescendo and Leangain methods.

Weekly fasting: This is another very popular style that is sometimes referred to as alternate-day fasting and involves a full 24 hours spent fasting or not fasting. Occasionally, these days are lumped together for 48 hours of fasting, but more commonly they alternate throughout the week. The 5:2 approach, where one fasts two days a week and does not fast the other five, is an example of this. On fasting days, individuals consume either no calories or limit intake to a mere 25 percent of daily caloric needs. On non-fasting days, they may resume their typical food intake. Many adopt this style of fasting after starting with time-restricted feeding.

Extended fasting: The most extreme and less common version of fasting, this method involves going a prolonged period before returning to normal food consumption. This kind (a.k.a. "long fasts") involves consuming less than 25 percent of caloric needs for at least 48 hours and up to a full week. This version is more suitable for those with a high level of social support who are seeking to positively shake up their lifestyle or obtain drastic results.

How it works

Healthy diets are typically associated with how much to eat, what foods to eat, and what foods to limit. We are constantly faced with "What should I eat?" Wouldn't it be a relief to spend less mental energy making choices that might promote stress and guilty feelings? In forgoing complicated diets centered around restricting food choices and portions, you can find peace by eating according to the clock. Fasting diets, regardless of the method, are based on periods of time when no calories are consumed. These fasting periods can range from 12 hours to over two days. Before we get into how to choose the fast best for your lifestyle demands and health goals, let's look at the major ways your body beneficially responds to fasting, including acute stress management, improved fat utilization, lean tissue preservation, and increased sensitivity to hunger hormones.

Your body will typically enter a fasted state after 8 to 12 hours, and you will begin to experience fasting's benefits.

First, this time period without food allows the gastric system to fully digest the last meal. Once that meal is completely digested, your stomach can take a food-processing break. This allows blood flow to be directed away from the gut to the brain and muscles to enhance mental focus and physical energy.

Second, not getting food as your body expects forces it to respond to that acute stress. This short-lived stress is actually very beneficial because it requires your body to react and respond, coming back stronger and healthier each time. Chronic stress is different. This harmful, long-term stress happens when the body is overwhelmed and unable to respond to acute stress. According to a 2013 study, enhancing the body's ability to cope with acute stress is part of what promotes physiological benefits of fasting.

As the fasting period continues, you run out of the body's preferred energy source: glucose. As you reach the 10- to 12-hour mark and your body depletes its readily available glucose, it is forced to tap into stored fat for energy production. Using stored fat has many upsides, including that it is a much slower and more intensive metabolic process to use fat for energy than glucose. To better utilize fat during a fasting period, cholesterol production decreases and fat storage is limited by the enzymatic activation. Fat utilization is just one internal benefit of fasting.

At first, this transition might trigger mild headaches, irritability, and fatigue as the body adjusts to utilizing fat for energy and hormones adjust to the body's current state. When food is withheld, ghrelin production is stimulated, causing feelings of increased hunger. In traditional diets, this works against your weight loss attempts because more ghrelin is associated with cravings, increased fat storage, and a decreased ability to maintain willpower. However, in fasting, the cycling of on/off eating periods doesn't excite long-term effects of chronic hunger or starvation. The body quickly adapts to being more sensitive to regulating these appetite hormones according to the fast/fed state. This regulation sensitivity includes secreting human growth hormone (HGH), which ramps up to break down fat for energy and promotes building lean tissue while reducing fat cell accumulation. HGH is suppressed during feeding periods and increased during fasting to preserve lean tissue. One 2003 study showed that HGH levels increase 50 to 2,000 percent during a fast. Women's bodies have been shown to release additional leptin and adiponectin to counteract ghrelin. When the body is fed again, leptin levels increase, signaling that the body is full. When you consistently fast, the on/off cycle improves the signaling of appetite hormones. Basically, consistent fasting helps your body maintain lean tissue and makes fat loss easier because the body becomes more sensitive and better able to respond to fast/fed changes.

Diets that require constant meals and snacks at all hours do not stimulate the same responses and you'll become blunted to what real hunger and satiety feel like, which leads to mindless eating, depressing portion control, and restrictive, unsustainable diets.

When exposed to a prolonged fast, the body begins a tissue rejuvenation process called autophagy, essentially using up old cells and replacing them with newer, healthier ones. Essentially, it is a process of stimulating natural cleansing and detoxing of cells.

Of course, the body is a very complex system and many lifestyle and biological internal factors are at play throughout the fasted and fed periods that vary greatly from person to person. The general synopsis is that fasting might be responsible for improved health outcomes and triggers reactions in the body that do not get stimulated when the body is constantly fed.

Understanding how exactly intermittent fasting work is one of the essential elements that need to be covered before you dive into it and start adopting this method of eating in your own life. By learning more about how it works, you can get a better idea of whether or not this might be a good option for you – and if you would be able to benefit from it truly.

This eating habit basically involves cycles of eating and abstaining from food. There are different techniques and methods that have been introduced over the last few years, so not everyone will follow this lifestyle option in the same way as others. Generally, however, all options that are available involved periods of time where food is consumed, and then periods where the person would completely avoid eating any type of food.

When eating normally, with three meals a day and in-between snacks, the body uses energy from the recently consumed meal first, seeking out carbohydrates (CHO) and sugars, which it prefers to burn before anything else. Without intermittent fasting, normal persons (non-diabetics) insulin sensitivity will be at normal levels, and will detect stored glycogen at "full level." With sufficient blood glucose levels, excess energy will be stored as fat. If this happens on a regular basis, the determinants for the difference in body weight will lie in the level of activity and metabolic rate which slows down with age, resulting in weight gain.

When on intermittent fasting, the body behaves differently when food is present (feasting) and during the period of abstinence (fasting), as compared to normal eating. The body produces insulin in response to the presence of food, enabling the body to get the most from them, maximizing nutrients for optimum results. Since eating is confined to a desired set window of 4, 6, or 8 hours, the body will not have a ready source of energy during the fasted state and will tend to extract energy from stored fat rather than from glucose traveling in the blood or glycogen stored in the liver or muscles.

Insulin sensitivity is increased after a fast. We can illustrate this insulin sensitivity by analyzing the cascade of events that take place when such a person eats something. As blood glucose rises, it activates a feedback mechanism which signals the pancreas to send insulin to the site where it is needed. An immediate response serves to lower the blood glucose and prevent its accumulation in the blood, or hyperglycemia. Here, insulin responds with a "now you see it, now you don't" type of mechanism: a sharp peak in response to the rising blood glucose, followed by an immediate decline. This is documented by lower readings of 2-hour postprandial blood glucose and insulin measurements.

Diabetics, on the other hand, suffer from insulin resistance, wherein the pancreas secretes only small bursts of insulin in response to glucose, followed by a slowed decline, resulting in higher 2-hour postprandial blood glucose and insulin measurements.

What Is the Purpose of Fasting?

For many centuries, people have fasted. Often, fasting was done because there was no food available to consume. In other situations, it was part of a religious belief. Moreover, many animals, including humans, fast when they fall sick. Thus, fasting is a standard process, as the body can handle extended periods of time without eating anything.

However, with fasting, there are specific changes in the body so that the body can counter the lack of nutrition in that particular fasting period. This is linked to cellular repair operations, genes, and hormones. During fasting, there is a significant decrease in insulin and blood sugar levels, and a radical elevation in growth hormones.

Thus, many people practice intermittent fasting to promote weight loss, as it is one of the simplest techniques to burn fat and restrict calories. Many also follow such techniques to improve their metabolism, as fasting can regulate various health markers and risk factors. In addition, intermittent fasting has been noted to help an individual live for a longer time. This has been proven through research conducted upon rodents, which had extended lifespans after a restriction in their calorie intake.

Another prominent benefit of IF is that it can help protect the body from diseases, such as Alzheimer's disease, cancer, type 2 diabetes, heart disease, etc. Many people who practice this fasting technique do it to lose weight and do not realize that it is also benefitting them clinically.

Thus, you can consider intermittent fasting to be an essential process for regulating your body weight and health simultaneously. With fewer meals, you have a better chance of living a healthy life. In addition, when you do not have to prepare extra dishes every day (because you are skipping meals), you can save a lot of time for other activities.

Chapter 2: History and Benefits of Fasting

A Brief History of Fasting

There is no point in the known human history wherein the concept of fasting has not existed in some shape or form. The voluntary act of abstaining from eating or drinking has deep roots in different cultures and religions around the world. Each type may vary at some point or another, but the core principles of fasting remain the same.

Fasting is as old as humanity, much older than any other type of diet. Ancient civilizations, like the Greeks, have recognized the intrinsic benefit of periodic fasting. These were often referred to as cycles of treatment, purification, and detox. Almost every culture and religion on earth perform certain fasting rituals.

Before the introduction of agriculture, people never eat three meals a day plus snacks. We only ate when we found food that could be separated by hours or days. Thus, from an evolutionary point of view, eating three meals a day is not a survival requirement. Perhaps, as a species, we would not have survived.

We have all forgotten this ancient practice before the 21st century. Fasting is bad for business, after all! Food producers allow us to eat snacks and multiple meals a day. Nutrition authorities warn against the severe effects of skip single meal. These messages have been drilled in our heads over time.

Even the motivations behind each variation tend to be of similar natures. For some, fasting is a way to heal the body and the mind. Most religions, on the other hand, believe it is way of strengthening the spirit and one's connection to a divine being.

To better illustrate the universality of fasting across time and location, here are the important historical highlights that would give you a better picture of the practice of fasting across different cultures and religions.

One of the earliest records of fasting show that a number of prominent ancient Greek figures were believers. For example, Pythagoras, a legendary Greek philosopher and mathematician, followed a 40-day starvation cycle in order to enhance his creativity and mental clarity.

The father of modern medicine, Hippocrates, was among the first to recognize the applications of fasting to the medical field. His observations of the human body had led him to a conclusion that a sick body would benefit from the absence of food.

Ancient Greek healers had also observed that the frequency of epileptic seizures was lower among patients who were engaging in a fast at the time compared those who were not.

Some ancient cultures, such as the Natives from North America, believed that fasting before a war would ensure their success in battle. They had also engaged in fasting to prevent the occurrence of wide-scale catastrophes like famine and drought.

Both the Old Testament and the New Testament of the Bible mention several instances of fasting. Even Jesus Christ himself had fasted for 40 days and 40 nights in a desert. Other Biblical figures who have also fasted include Moses, Elijah, and Paul, one of Jesus' apostles.

Given its presence in the Bible, the Christian church encourages its followers to participate in a 40-day fast before Easter as a form of repentance. Though the exact date on which this practice had first been adapted is unknown, the fasting guidelines imposed among Christians have become more lenient throughout the years.

Muslims practice fasting since it is one of the Five Pillars of Islam—the others being (1) pilgrimage, (2) prayer, (3) declaration of faith, and (4) charity. They believe that through fasting, they would become closer to Allah become it begins with a spiritual intention. Furthermore, fasting fosters solidarity among Muslims who are also fasting, and amplifies feelings of compassion and empathy towards those who are suffering.

These beliefs culminate during Ramadan, a Muslim holiday that is characterized by a month-long period of fasting. During this time, all Muslims are prohibited from consuming food while there is daylight.

Buddhist monks and nuns abide by the rules of Vinyana, wherein it is stated that followers should not eat anything after they had taken their meals at noon. However, the followers themselves do not consider this as a form of fasting. Instead, they think of it as a part of their normal routine.

The fasting days among Hindus differ depending on which deity they are following. For example, Vishnu requires fasting on a Thursday, while followers of Shiva fast on a Monday. Hindus also engage in monthly fasting periods that occur after certain lunar phases.

There are also individuals who perform complete or partial fasting as part of a religious practice called Vratas. Aside from abstaining from food and/or water, those who are practicing it are required to observe personal hygiene, celibacy, and honesty, among others.

The traditional form of Judaism includes a requirement of 6 fasting days within a given year among its followers. The fasting day lasts from sunset of a particular day up to the sunset of the succeeding day.

Jains believe that fasting regulates the demands of their bodies, eliminates their accumulated bad karma, and rejuvenates their spirits. As such, they make it a point to incorporate fasting into their day to day lives. Aside from abstaining from food and water, Jains are also required to worship their gods, serve Jain monks and nuns, and engage in acts of charity while fasting.

A secular fasting holiday in Geneva, Switzerland called the "Jeune Genevois" originated in the Middle Ages. During that period, the people dedicated certain days of the year for fasting as a form of penitence whenever they experienced epidemics, wars, and other big-scale calamities.

As shown through these examples of fasting traditions, fasting had been in existence for hundreds of years, and will continue to be practiced across the world in the foreseeable future.

Fasting has also undergone evolution throughout the years. Though most practitioners perform it as a part of their religious beliefs, a growing number of health enthusiasts have recognized the benefits of fasting on their health.

If you are not fasting due to your religion, then you may still practice fasting according to your current lifestyle, personal preferences, and fitness goals. To guide you through this, the next section of this book covers the various modern ways of fasting that you may consider doing.

Benefits of fasting

A number of studies, like those mentioned above, have been done on both humans and animals. These studies evaluated the many benefits of intermittent fasting for controlling weight and other bodily functions. The results have been phenomenal.

Some of the popular health benefits of the IF regimen are:

• Weight loss: This is the most common health benefit that you can achieve through the intermittent fasting method. You can reduce your belly fat and weight without compromising the calorie intake.

• Insulin resistance: IF is also capable of decreasing insulin resistance in the body. A follower of this fasting technique will witness a decrease in the levels of insulin by an impressive 20 to 31%. Furthermore, IF reduces the blood sugar levels up to 6%. These figures are enough to protect a person from type 2 diabetes.

- Inflammation: Much research has revealed a decrease in inflammation markers, which have been noted to be significant catalysts for several chronic diseases.

- Cardiovascular health: IF is known to decrease bad cholesterol levels (LDL) and promote HDL or good cholesterol. In addition, it may decrease the presence of blood triglycerides, which is one of the causes of cardiovascular diseases.

- Cancer: Animals on the IF diet have shown results that display cancer prevention abilities.

- Brain function: IF improves brain function by promoting the growth of nerve cells. Thus, it can help protect against neural disorders, such as Alzheimer's disease.

- Anti-aging properties: IF has been noted to promote longevity in rats, which were part of a fasting experiment. It was found that rats following this diet lived up to 83% longer than rats that weren't on the diet.

Note that while IF may have health benefits, the experiments are still at an initial stage. Several of these studies were conducted for a short duration upon various animals. Therefore, there are still many unanswered questions.

Impact of Intermittent Fasting on Lifestyle

While eating healthy is a simple process, it is not as easy as it seems. One of its primary hurdles is the work needed to cook healthy recipes. However, it does save time by reducing the workload required to prepare several meals a day, thus letting you spend your time doing other things. This makes IF a popular choice among people who prefer life hacks to make their lives easier and healthier. In this way, IF has a significant impact on the lifestyle of an individual.

Intermittent Fasting: Mental Advantages

In addition to physical benefits, IF has mental benefits. This diet plan offers significant benefits related to:

- Boosting memory

- Shielding the mind from neurological disorders such as epilepsy and Alzheimer's disease

- Improving mental focus and clarity

Intermittent Fasting: Enhancing Cognitive Function and Reducing Stress

Intermittent fasting has also shown significant effects with respect to the brain and memory. People who have practiced this diet plan were better able to retain their ability to learn, decreased their oxidative stress, and enhanced their memory.

Many researchers say that this activity takes place because this fasting program manipulates the brain cells to perform more efficiently. During fasting, the cells undergo low/moderate stress, which is why the most efficient cells among them start improvising and adapting to the new condition. This way, the weak cells die, but the stronger ones survive and improve the abilities of the brain.

You can compare it to a high-intensity workout routine at the gym. Exercising is also a type of physical stress that forces your body to endure uncomfortable conditions. As you progress with the regimen, your body starts to adapt to the new conditions, building your muscles, stamina, etc. However, you must rest between your workouts to keep your body ready for the next session.

A similar approach exists when you are practicing IF. Here, your resting intervals will comprise healthy and regular eating sessions, balanced with fasting sessions. That way, you can benefit both your mind and your body.

Thus, you can see that intermittent fasting is capable of improving your cognitive operations due to moderate stress at a cellular level to support and sculpt you.

Additional Benefits of Intermittent Fasting

If you are planning to try intermittent fasting, you will experience the following benefits. Remember that these results will come about only when you are following a strict fasting and eating regimen. IF will help your body achieve the following benefits:

Improves fat loss

If you follow the 16/8 method in which you eat within an eight-hour period and fast for the remaining 16 hours, you can lose a significant amount of weight without having to worry about calories. No doubt, this method will cause the body to lose weight, but those who follow a healthy diet will be able to achieve two times the weight loss twice than those who prefer junk food achieve. Thus, through intermittent fasting, you have a way to accomplish your goals, but only when you follow it healthily.

Increases muscle mass

Many people believe that their muscles will fade away while fasting. However, as per research, a 24-hour fast elevated the growth hormone in humans (HGH) up to 1300% for women and 2000% for men. HGH is known for its significance in building muscle cells. With such high numbers, there is a huge effect on the physique of an individual following IF. Increased HGH levels offer enhanced bone mass, increased body mass, and reduced body fat.

Faster recovery

Increased HGH also helps synthesize protein that causes the body to repair and heal faster after an injury or workout session.

Adds suppleness to the skin

With an increase in age, HGH levels decrease. However, during a study, participants who were provided with HGH supplements were found to build muscle and lose fat at a much higher rate. In addition, their skin improved in strength, making it more resistant to wrinkles and sagging.

Reduces the rate of aging

With fasting, your body starts producing stem cells at a much faster rate. These stem cells can be manipulated to become any cell in the body. Therefore, they can replace damaged and old cells, keeping your body younger at the cellular level. These stem cells can help with chronic pain, old injuries, joints, skin, etc.

Therefore, instead of going for stem cell therapy, which can be costly, your other option is to focus on intermittent fasting.

Enhances brain functions

Through fasting, you can improve your brain. When you fast, your brain starts generating a protein known as BNF, which is a very crucial building block. This protein helps improve memory and learning power.

In addition, it helps develop complex and robust neural networks to keep the brain functioning smoothly and speedily. This is necessary to keep the brain functions active as you get older.

Triggers autophagy

This process may sound cruel for the cells in your body, but it is of crucial importance. New and strong cells eat away damaged and old cells to make space for fresh and strong ones. This is like a tune-up operation for your body; it will keep the body running smoothly and promote longevity. Through intermittent fasting, the process of autophagy can be triggered.

Reduces inflammation

IF reduces inflammation markers and oxidative stress. Inflammation is responsible for diseases, aging, and poor performance of the body, which is why it must be reduced or eliminated. Preventing inflammation will help the body function more efficiently with increased longevity. IF offers you an upgrade that helps your body adapt to new and tougher conditions, ultimately enhancing your resistance and endurance for your eating habits. The result is a stronger, more efficient body that works on less energy.

☐   Heart health

Heart disease is the leading cause of death worldwide

High blood pressure, high LDL cholesterol, and high triglyceride concentrations are among the leading risk factors for cardiovascular disease.

One study involving 16 men and women with obesity showed that intermittent fasting reduced blood pressure by 6% in just eight weeks.

In the same study, it was also found that intermittent fasting lowers LDL cholesterol by 25% and triglycerides by 32%.

However, data on the relationship between intermittent fasting and increased levels of LDL cholesterol and triglycerides do not agree.

A study with 40 people with normal weight showed that four weeks of intermittent fasting during the Islamic holiday of Ramadan does not lead to a decrease in LDL cholesterol or triglycerides.

Better studies with more reliable methods are needed before researchers can fully understand the effect of intermittent fasting on heart health.

☐ Diabetes

Intermittent fasting can also effectively help manage and reduce the risk of developing diabetes.

Like constant calorie restriction, intermittent fasting seems to reduce certain risk factors for diabetes.

This is mainly due to a decrease in insulin levels and a decrease in insulin resistance.

However, intermittent fasting may not be as beneficial for women as it is for men in terms of blood sugar levels.

A small study showed that blood sugar control worsened in women after a 22-day fast, while men did not hurt blood sugar levels.

Despite this side effect, a decrease in insulin resistance and insulin resistance is likely to reduce the risk of developing diabetes, especially for people with pre-diabetes.

☐　　Weight loss

Intermittent fasting can be a simple and effective way to lose weight if done correctly, as regular short-term posts can help you consume fewer calories and lose pounds.

A review of studies conducted in 2018 for overweight adults showed that intermittent fasting resulted in an average weight loss of 15 pounds (6.8 kg) for 3–12 months.

Another review showed that intermittent fasting reduced body weight by 3–8% in adults with overweight or obesity for 3–24 weeks. The survey also showed that participants reduced waist size by 3–7% over the same period.

It should be noted that the long-term effect of intermittent fasting on weight loss in women remains to be seen.

In the short term, intermittent hunger seems to help in weight loss. However, the amount you lose is likely to depend on the number of calories you consume during periods without fasting, and how long you keep your lifestyle.

☐   It can help you eat less

Going to intermittent fasting can, of course, help you eat less.

One study found that young people ate 650 calories less per day when their food intake was limited to a four-hour interval.

Another study conducted on 24 healthy men and women was devoted to studying the effect of a long 36-hour fast on eating habits. Despite the consumption of extra calories in post-post day, participants reduced the total calorie balance by 1,900 calories, which is a significant reduction.

Other health benefits

Several studies carried out in humans and animals suggest that intermittent fasting may bring other health benefits.

Reducing inflammation: Some studies show that intermittent fasting can reduce key inflammatory markers. Chronic inflammation can lead to weight gain and various health problems.

Improving mental well-being: one study found those eight weeks of intermittent fasting reduced depression and overeating, improving body image in obese adults.

Increased life expectancy: intermittent fasting has been shown to increase life expectancy in rats and mice by 33–83%. The effect on life expectancy in humans remains to be determined.

Preserving Muscle Mass: Intermittent fasting seems to be more effective for maintaining muscle mass compared to constant calorie restriction. Large muscle mass helps you burn more calories, even at rest

In particular, the health benefits of intermittent fasting for women should be more carefully studied in well-designed studies in humans before any conclusions can be drawn.

Chapter 3: What is Intermittent Fasting?

Intermittent fasting (IF) describes the eating pattern that runs between the periods of fasting and normal eating.

The most common methods include fasting every other day, daily 16-hour fasting, or fasting for 24 hours, two days a week. For this guide, the term intermittent fasting will be used to describe all modes.

It can also help reduce the risk of heart disease and diabetes, preserve muscle mass, and improve psychological well-being.

Moreover, this diet can help save time in the kitchen since you have fewer meals to plan, cook, and cook.

For these reasons, women should consider a modified approach to intermittent fasting, for example, shorter periods of fasting and fewer fasting days.

Intermittent fasting is different from the usual diet plan that focuses on the caloric content or macronutrient type of your food choices. It focuses more on when you can eat to create the effects that it can cause to your body. Instead, intermittent fasting would have you follow a dieting pattern involving alternating phases of fasting and eating.

During the fasting phase, you are restricted from eating anything that contains calories. It is only during the eating phase that you can consume food or drink containing calories.

Contrary to popular belief, intermittent fasting alone does not directly cause weight loss. It is still caused by the caloric deficit, which is brought about by the fewer meals that arise from the limited time you have for eating. However, unlike diets that solely rely on caloric deficit, it is more sustainable in the long term, more satisfying, and more flexible.

This focus on when you eat your food instead of what you eat gives intermittent fasting its simplicity. You do not have to count calories for every meal. You do not have to restrict your food choices. And, you do not have to follow a meal plan with stringent macronutrient portions.

Determining Who Can Benefit from Intermittent Fasting

Intermittent fasting is not a diet. You may be tired of trying anything with the word "diet" in it when it comes to losing those extra pounds. Intermittent Fasting is a way to lose weight that involves a structured program of when you should eat and when you should not eat. You will be able to create your own plan that will suit your needs, especially if you can go through with it quickly for a whole day! Quick means spending twelve full hours empty before a meal. You can increase your fasting time later when the program continues.

If you have been attempting to lose weight, you probably have tried diets like the Atkins diet which is based on the frequent eating theory. Those who advocate such diets advise you to eat often throughout the day. The idea behind those food plans is to make your metabolism work faster only by eating more. The quicker your metabolism, the faster you will lose weight. However, the more food you ate, the more you wished to eat, and the more your weight was left intact. If you decide to enroll in an intermittent program, your meal frequency will have to be reduced. You will have to do without breakfast sometimes.

You probably sleep 6 to 8 hours. Your body is in fasting mode during this time. When your body is fasting, it generates more insulin. More insulin in your body increases your sensitivity to insulin. If your organism is more sensitive to insulin, you lose more fat. The brilliance of the intermittent weight loss program is that you spend your breakfast on extending the insulin sensitivity of your body. This means that your body will be losing fat for a long time which translates into losing more weight.

A more extended fasting mode also has a great effect on your body's hormone levels. Your body produces growth hormones by skipping breakfast or eating at a specific time. Producing growth hormone is essential when you are trying to lose weight because it helps your body to do this exact task. If your weight loss program is intermittent, your growth hormone levels are usually at their highest which results in losing more weight. High levels of growth hormone also have several other health benefits in your body. This program is just excellent!

Fasting is highly recommended for anyone who wishes to live a longer and healthier life. Many medical experts also recognize this as an excellent way to manage and reverse several chronic health conditions, such as heart diseases and cancer. However, studies show that fasting may not be effective for all types of people.

As with any major health decision that you have to make, it is best to seek first the professional opinion of your physician before committing yourself to significant changes in your lifestyle and diet. Fasting may aggravate any existing health condition, especially the ones that you may not be aware of at this point.

Have an open discussion with your doctor about your goals for fasting, as well as the probable side-effects this activity could have on your health. By doing so, you would be able to engage in fasting without any serious reservations about your wellbeing.

For your reference, here is a rundown of specific groups of people, and their respective likelihood of benefiting from fasting:

Children

Average children, up to the age of 18, are not recommended to fast. At most, health experts may advise parents to control the frequency of their child's meals throughout the day. Children should not be abstaining from food for long periods of time. The nutrition they gain from their meals are essential for their growth and development.

Even overweight children are not exempted from this. Parents, with the guidance of the child's pediatrician or a nutritionist, should try restructuring first the child's diet. The objective for such a move is to prevent the child from consuming junk food and too much sugar, and replace them with healthier options.

Once the overweight child begins eating a well-balanced diet, most parents do not have any reason left to wonder if child has to go through a fast to lose the excess weight.

If you still think that a child below the age of 18 would benefit from a fast, you should consult with the child's physician first.

Healthy Adults

Being in good health does not exclude healthy adults from benefiting from fasting. In fact, going into a fast from time to time may be helpful in sustaining their current health condition.

High-Level Athletes

Several benefits of fasting are attractive for many athletes. Fasting enables the body to recover faster from being strained, and it improves the absorption of nutrients of the digestive system. Both benefits are critical in the process of developing muscles and increasing physical strength.

Athletes should take extra care when adapting fasting into their normal routines. Experts do not suggest going on a fast right before and during game days. Fasting should not also be done when the athlete has to engage in intense and extended practice sessions. Doing any of these would seriously deplete them to the point that the continual act of abstaining from food becomes harmful to their health.

Pregnant Women

Multiple studies have been conducted on the effects of fasting among pregnant Muslim women during Ramadan. To date, researchers have found that fasting has no negative effects on the mother or the child.

Pregnancy, however, is a highly sensitive state, so pregnant women are encouraged to get the approval of their respective doctors first before entering a fast.

Vegetarians or Vegans

Fasting is compatible with almost every type of lifestyle or diet. Due to the dietary restrictions of vegetarians and vegans, the effects of fasting may even be enhanced when implemented properly.

Individuals with Type-2 Diabetes

Fasting has long been used by medical experts as a method of reversing Type-2 Diabetes. Various research studies on this strategy show consistent results indicating the positive effects of fasting to diabetic people. Still, if you are diabetic too, you should consult first with your doctor before adapting any form of fasting.

Individuals who are Immunosuppressed

People who are suffering from HIV, AIDS, lupus, different types of cancer, or any similar disorders related to the immune system should seek the opinion of their physicians before making any major lifestyle or dietary changes, such as fasting.

Though fasting is largely beneficial to most people, it may wreak havoc to the delicate balance of bodily chemicals and processes of an immunosuppressed individual.

Individuals with Eating Disorders

An eating disorder is rooted upon the physical, mental, and emotional aspects of a person suffering from it. Therefore, there is no guarantee that fasting may help resolve these food-related issues. Those who have been diagnosed with eating disorders should get the approval of their psychotherapists first before applying the principles of fasting into their lives.

As you can see, almost every group of people may benefit from fasting. However, most groups are also encouraged to get the opinion of medical experts prior to making a commitment to fasting.

In case you want to do a preliminary self-assessment before your consultation, here is a set of guide questions that you may reflect upon to determine whether or not fasting is for you.

How well do handle hunger pangs?

Can you fully commit to fasting for at least three months?

Do you think you have the physical and mental fortitude to last through an entire fasting period?

How would you describe your current diet?

How would you describe your current lifestyle?

How do you regard the thought of having to exercise regularly?

Do you have support system who can motivate you and hold you accountable while you are fasting?

It is best if you would write down your answers to these questions in a personal journal. Refer to your responses before making a final decision regarding fasting. Even if your physician has given you clearance to pursue with this, you must be willing to commit yourself, and go through the highs and lows of fasting as best you can.

Take the time to reflect upon the questions given above. Doing so would help you figure out if you have what it takes to reap the numerous benefits of fasting.

It is also worth mentioning the groups of people that shouldn't fast intermittently:

• Women who are pregnant or breastfeeding, unless they are allowed to do so by their doctors.

• Those who are underweight and malnourished.

• Children under 18 and elders.

• Those with gout.

• Those that have Gastroesophageal reflux (GERD) disease.

• Those with eating disorders should consult their physicians first.

• Diabetes and insulin patients must contact their physicians in advance, as dosages must be through.

• The drug consumers must consult their physicians first as the timing of medicines may be affected.

• Those with high stress or cortisol issues should not be rapid since fasting is another stressor.

• Those who train very hard most days of the week.

When to Avoid Intermittent Fasting as a Woman

While intermittent fasting is flexible, versatile, and adaptable to many different lifestyles, it is still the case that many women should probably **not** attempt IF, for the sake of their overall health. Chapters 7, 8, 9, & 10 will go on to discuss four additional types of women that should be especially cautious proceeding with intermittent fasting, but still, for these women, things **can** be productive when practiced the correct way. Conversely, there are a handful of types of women that aren't well-suited to intermittent fasting in any fashion, for the sake of their lives or others, and this chapter is dedicated to these women.

The following pages will address five different profiles of candidates who wouldn't be conducive to growing and healing with the intermittent fasting meal plan. Of course, the sex distinction in our studies of intermittent fasting plays a huge role in this chapter, for the intersections of sex and disease or disorder are what makes these candidates so problematic about IF itself. From the pregnant candidate to the underweight woman, the female patient with the eating disorder, the female diabetic, and the woman with the troubling personality, it remains true that intermittent fasting isn't necessarily for everyone.

However, even with these limitations in place, there is lingering potential for each of these types of women to come to a place of progress or healing eventually that would allow them to move through their struggles and attempt IF at their own pace. Therefore, if you qualify as any of the following candidates, don't be too dejected or hopeless! With the appropriate personal growth and the right lessons being presented to you, you'll surely come back to intermittent fasting as soon as you're ready for it.

Exploring the Pregnant Candidate

Although intermittent fasting can give you increased energy, better metabolism, and stronger cellular protection, the risks clearly outweigh the benefits for pregnant IF candidates. Since the female body is made to bear children, the effects of intermittent fasting are already debated in their relation to female health, but when it comes to pregnant and soon-to-be mothers, the answer to the question is a clear "No." Pregnant women should not be working with intermittent fasting.

For the expecting mother, long periods between meals are not necessarily such a good thing. The pregnant woman will need to be eating whenever she's hungry to gain the weight and nutrients her future child will need to survive. Furthermore, she will need to combat the morning sickness and nausea that go along with pregnancy, and if she's concerned about her timing with the intermittent fast, she might put herself in a detrimental situation for her overall health by mistake.

If you're recently pregnant but had used intermittent fasting previously with great success, you can shift back to focusing on **what** you eat rather than **when** you eat. Just as it is for the standard person shifting from normal eating to intermittent fasting and going from **what**'s eaten to **when** it's eaten, when you switch from IF to pregnancy, you'll shift eating habits once again. This time, however, you'll try to make sure you're eating the best foods whenever possible; not just in your okayed eating windows.

If you're having trouble stopping your intermittent fast while you've just become pregnant, you might want to reconsider the reasons behind your IF in the first place. Is it really for your health, or does it support your controlling tendency to limit your weight? Try to make sure that when you're pregnant, you're looking for what supports your health, rather than your mental image of what you should look like and what you think you should weigh. Pregnancy is a beautiful time, but it's not about restriction, it's about abundance and weight gain and growth, so it doesn't mesh well with IF at all.

Exploring the Underweight Candidate

For women who are already underweight, intermittent fasting might not be the best thing for your health. Surely, there are unintentionally underweight women who don't have the time they'd like to have for eating or who don't have the energy they'd like to have for cooking, but there are also intentionally underweight women who are looking for an additional method to use to keep off that "excess" weight for good.

If you're incredibly underweight already (even if you don't feel like it!), steer clear of intermittent fasting. If you're only five to ten pounds underweight and you're seeking spiritual enlightenment, lessened brain fog, or a jolt to your digestive system, IF may work just fine for you without being problematic. (While you **might** find a method of IF that works alright for you in this case, don't make the hard and fast decisions on eating pattern switching without first making sure to consult a doctor or health professional.)

Essentially, the problem arises when the individual is already over 10 pounds underweight, for these individuals aren't giving their digestive systems a break or a free moment for healing by switching to IF. Instead, the individual in this stance forces his or her digestive system to claw at itself and scrape at the bottom of the barrel to try and heal itself. I shouldn't have to explain why that simply **won't work**.

Overall, something you can use to determine whether you're in the healthy or unhealthy weight range is your BMI (Body Mass Index). If your BMI is anywhere between 18.5 and 25, you're in the healthy weight range. However, if you're lower than 18.5, be cautious about attempting intermittent fasting. If you're lower than 17, definitely do **not** try this method, for your body can't stand to lose anything else, and to choose IF would cause extreme detriment to your health rather than aid it.

Exploring the Candidate with an Eating Disorder

For the individual with an eating disorder, no matter what variety, intermittent fasting may seem to be helpful, but it will only function as a trigger for that person's disorder. No matter who you are, if you approach intermittent fasting for healing or weight loss, you're probably doing so because you want to switch from stuffing yourself of emptiness to healing yourself with goodness. Your focus, in other words, likely falls on growth (not physically but emotionally, spiritually, mentally, and regarding health capacity) rather than withering.

For the individual suffering from an eating disorder, all attempts toward health and growth are skewed by distortions of body image and self-esteem. Essentially, all attempts toward health and growth are twisted by the compulsory drive to purge. If you or someone you know struggled or struggles with anorexia, bulimia, orthorexia, binge eating, purging, avoidant/restrictive food intake disorder, or any other eating disorder, be extremely curious and demanding with them if they share an interest in intermittent fasting.

Question their inspirations and drives; demand they are honest with you. The likelihood is greater than not that this person is using intermittent fasting as a way to lose weight they can't afford to lose rather than to get healthier in general. If you're able to discern it at all, the individual's reason for **starting** IF is the best way to ascertain their true intentions. It can be hard to tell who has an eating disorder and who doesn't, but the way people talk about food, body image, fasting, and dieting can reveal more than you could ever anticipate. And once you **can** tell who has an eating disorder, help them stay clear from IF because it can really exacerbate their circumstances despite their (and your) best intentions.

Exploring the Diabetic Candidate

If you're already on insulin, as a diabetic most likely, you're already working to keep your levels of blood sugar at balance. If you add into the mix IF work to increase or decrease insulin resistance (to help with weight loss), you'll put yourself in a truly dangerous spot. People with diabetes should absolutely **not** skip doses of insulin to lose weight by lowering blood sugar. This would be disastrous for someone who has diabetes because they'd surely lose the weight, but they'd feel drained to a disastrous degree because humans do

need this sugar or glucose in our blood to derive energy.

So, if you have diabetes, stay away from intermittent fasting. It's unfortunate, I know, but this type of eating pattern change will do absolutely nothing good for you. As with the pregnant candidate, you could try to switch the foods you're eating instead of when you're eating. By adding the right, healthful foods into your diet, you might find that the weight that sticks to you so stubbornly can be depleted with your condition being made none the worse. However, be careful if you're diabetic when it comes to **fasting disguised as dieting**. If you feel inclined to try a juice or liquid diet, second guess those inclinations, for it's very likely that this type of diet would cause extra stress to your system, what with the high glycemic and fiber-free contents of some juices.

Basically, if you're diabetic and feeling inclined to make your life healthier, don't limit **when** you eat and don't just drink liquids. Rather than restricting whatsoever, try to **incorporate** healthier, more whole foods that are oriented towards healing innately and then maybe add exercise into the mix when you're ready for it.

Exploring Problematic Character Traits

While the previous entries in this chapter have to deal with physical traits and conditions, this final one has to do more so with personality and character attributes instead. The truth of the matter is that some personality types will not mesh well with the lifestyle connected to intermittent fasting. Whether you're controlling, OCD, impatient, moody, reserved, or just too young, you're not in for a "treat" by taking the first steps toward the intermittent fasting lifestyle. Nevertheless, the fact holds that if you can work through your struggles and face your (personality) demons, you might find yourself changed by intermittent fasting in ways no one would have ever expected.

Controlling people expect the world to be easily manipulated to suit their needs, urges, and comforts. Unfortunately, the world doesn't often act so easily shapeable, which puts controlling individuals in tough places. In fasting and dieting especially, control goes out the window and natural progress/timelines take its place. Therefore, controlling individuals might have trouble adjusting to intermittent fasting. Although these people will be able to make changes to their techniques as they go along, they still won't be able to actualize the changes they want with any immediacy. For controlling people, working with intermittent fasting will be a huge challenge, but it's definitely not impossible.

People who are impatient will also have a hard time with intermittent fasting because of what their expectations of the world happen to be. Impatient people expect the world to go fast, for things to be where they expect it **when** they expect it, and for progress to be made when they're ready for it to be made. In essence, impatient people are the opposite of productive intermittent fasters, for people skilled and practiced with IF know that patience is the ultimate virtue. It takes two weeks only to get fully past just the **detoxification** period for intermittent fasting, so clearly, impatient people will need those urges recalibrated before they're ready to handle the personal practice of consistency and waiting that gives life to the IF technique (and lifestyle).

Moody individuals will likely only see their emotional situations worsened by intermittent fasting, but these types of people often don't choose to fast intermittently because they want to fix their mood disorders. Instead, these people choose IF to lose weight, gain energy, fight aging, heal themselves or otherwise, and the emotional side-effects are just that. I recommend these individuals look at the bigger picture of intermittent fasting. This eating pattern and lifestyle change can make great waves in one's life that cause him or her to feel increasingly moody or troubled. By having increased awareness of the bigger picture, moody people might be able to hold off on transitioning to IF until they're healed enough to handle all the switch has to offer.

People who are excessively reserved or conservative in personality may find that intermittent fasting doesn't work for them because they struggle through the detox period and can't get any farther. It is true that the first two weeks of intermittent fasting – the detox period – are intense, both physically and emotionally. Sometimes, people break down into tears or have emotional explosions otherwise during this detoxification time, and overly reserved or conservative individuals will likely **not** appreciate being exposed to moments like this, much less that potential within their selves. If these types of people can learn to laugh at themselves and ride emotional waves more calmly, they'll have as much to gain from IF as any of the best of us.

Finally, when considering young people under the age of 18, we get back into physical traits and conditions a bit more than character traits, but it's undeniable that someone's youth makes it very difficult for intermittent fasting to work in his or her favor. No offense, but you're immature, and your body is even more immature, so you need all the available nutrients around you to help you grow properly. Limiting nutritional intake in any way (whether it's the **what** you eat or **when** it happens) will not be good for you until you're at least 18 and living your best life in that strong, fully-actualized, adult body.

Chapter 4: How Intermittent Fasting works?

Intermittent fasting is the technique of scheduling your meals for your body to obtain the most out of them. Instead of reducing your calorie usage in half, denying yourself of all the foods you appreciate, or diving into a classy diet plan trend, Intermittent fasting is a natural, rational, and healthy and balanced technique of eating that advertises weight loss. There are whole lots of means to approach intermittent fasting.

It's specified as a particular eating pattern. This technique concentrates on changing when you take in, as opposed to what you consume.

When you begin Intermittent fasting, you will certainly higher than likely to maintain your calorie.

Intake the same, however as opposed to spreading your meals throughout the day, you will certainly eat larger dishes throughout a shorter amount of time. Instead of eating 3 to 4 meals a day, you might consume one large meal at 11 am, after that an additional big meal at 6 pm, without any meal in between 11 am and 6 pm, and also after 6 pm, no meal up until 11 am the following day. This is just one strategy of recurring fasting, and also others will be described in this book in later phases.

You first must comprehend why this strategy functions. Intermittent Fasting is a method utilised by lots of bodybuilders, professional athletes, and physical fitness masters to keep their muscle mass high and their body fat percentage low. It is a primary method that allows you to eat the foods you take pleasure in, while still encouraging fat loss and muscle gain or upkeep. Intermittent fasting can be done short term or long term, but the very best outcomes originate from adopting this approach into your daily lifestyle.

The word "fasting" may worry the average person, Intermittent fasting does not relate to starving yourself. To comprehend the principals behind successful Intermittent fasting, we'll initially review the body's digestion state: the fed state and the fasting state.

For 3 to 5 hours after eating a meal, your body is in what is referred to as the "fed state." Throughout the fed state, your insulin levels increase to soak up and digest your meal. When your insulin levels are high, it is extremely difficult for your body to burn fat. Insulin is a hormone produced by the pancreas to manage glucose levels in the bloodstream. Its purpose is to control insulin is technically a storage hormonal agent. When insulin levels become so high, your body starts burning your food for energy rather than your saved fat which is why increased levels of it prevent weight loss.

After the 3 to 5 hours are up, your body has actually finished processing the meal, and you enter the post-absorptive state. The post-absorptive state lasts anywhere from 8 to 12 hours. When your body gets in, after this time space is the fasted state. Due to the fact that your body has actually completely processed your food by this. point, your insulin levels are reduced, making your stored fat incredibly available for shedding.

In the fasted state, your body has no food passed on used for power, so your conserved fat is melted rather. Recurring fasting enables your body to reach a sophisticated weight loss state that you would typically get to with the average ' 3 meals daily' eating pattern. This aspect alone is the factor that many individuals observe fast outcomes with Intermittent fasting without also making alterations to their workout routines, how a lot they consume, or what they consume. They are merely altering the timing as well as the pattern of their food intake. It might take some time to get when you begin an intermittent fasting program into the swing of things. Don't get discouraged! Simply get back if you slip up into your Intermittent fasting pattern when you can. Avoid beating yourself up, or feeling guilty. Negative self-talk will only lengthen you returning to your pattern.

Making a lifestyle change involves a deliberate effort, and nobody expects you to do it entirely right now. If you are not in the habit of going long periods without eating, intermittent fasting will take some getting used to. As long as you select the right technique for you, remain focused, and stay focused, you will master it in no time.

Unlike some of the other diet plans that you may undertake, the Intermittent fast is one that will work. It uses your body and how it works to its advantage in helping you to lose weight. When you hear, it is easy to get a bit afraid about fasting. You might assume that you need to spend weeks and days without eating (and who has the self-control to quit their food for that long even when they do want to reduce weight) and that it will be too tight for you.

Intermittent fasting is a bit various than you may think of. Not just is it tough to go on a fast for weeks at a time but it is also not good for the body. If you end up being on, your body will frequently go into starvation mode, the fast for too long. It assumes that you remain in time without much food and. The body will work on conserving the calories and assisting you to hold on to the fat and calories for as long as possible. This suggests that not only are you hungry, but you are likewise missing out on out on slimming down.

You do not have to get too worried about how this Intermittent fast will work in the hunger mode. The Intermittent fast is efficient because you are not going to fast for so long that the body enters into this starvation mode and stops reducing weight. Rather, it will make the fast persist long enough that you will be able to speed up the metabolic process.

With the Intermittent fast, you will discover that when you opt for a couple of hours without eating (normally no more than 2 - 4 hours), the body is not going to go right into starvation mode. Instead, it is going to consume the calories that are readily available. If you eat the right quantity of calories for the day, the body is going to revert to making use of the stored reserves of fat and use it as energy. As such, when following an intermittent fasting plan, you force your body to burn more fat without putting in any additional work.

Here are a few fast suggestions for success:

Primarily, it is essential not to expect to see results from your new way of life immediately. Instead, you need to focus on devoting to the process for a minimum of 30 days before you can start to judge the outcomes precisely.

Second, it is vital to remember that the high quality of the food you place into your body still matters as it will certainly simply take a few fast food meals to reverse all of your hard job.

For the ideal outcomes, you will intend to include in a light exercise regimen during quick days as well as a much more basic routine for full-calorie days.

Intermittent Fasting refers to nutritional consuming patterns that include not consuming or badly restricting calories for a long term time period, periodic Fasting

There are different subgroups of periodic fasting each with individual variation in the period of the rapid; some for hrs, others for day(s). This has ended up being an extremely preferred topic in the scientific research community as a result of every one of the prospective benefits on physical fitness as well as wellness that are being discovered. How The Process Works

If you are seeking to lose a significant amount of weight, then you are going to have to have a look at your diet plan more closely, but if you want to lose a few pounds for the beach, then you might find that a couple of weeks of Intermittent fasting can do that for you.

While fasting , it is advisable to drink plenty of water to avoid tea, coffee and dehydration are okay as long as you take a splash of milk. If you can handle it, then it would be best to stick to the coffee, water, and tea.

Whatever your diet plan is whether it's healthy or not you ought to see weight reduction after about 3 weeks of Intermittent fasting and do not be dissuaded if you don't discover much development initially, it's not a race and its much better to drop weight in a direct style over time rather than crash losing a few pounds which you will put straight back on. After the first month, you may wish to have a look at your diet on non-fasting days and eliminate high sugar foods and any scrap that you may usually consume. I have found that intermittent fasting over the long term tends to make me wish to consume more healthy foods as a natural routine.

If you are practising intermittent fasting for bodybuilding then you may wish to consider taking a look at your macro-nutrients and exercising just how much protein and carbohydrate you require to consume, this is much more complex, and you can discover information about this on several sites which you will need to hang around investigating for the best outcomes. There are lots of advantages to intermittent fasting, which you will see as you progress, a few of these advantages consist of more energy, less bloating, a clearer mind, and a general sensation of wellness. It's crucial not to succumb to any temptation to binge eat after a fasting duration, as this will negate the impact gained from the intermittent fasting period.

So in conclusion just by following a twice a week 24-hour intermittent fasting strategy for a few weeks you will slim down however if you can enhance your diet plan on the days that you do not fast then you will lose more weight and if you can stay with this system, then you will keep the weight off without turning to any fad diet or diet plans that are difficult to adhere to.

Chapter 5: Impact of Intermittent Fasting on your body

How Intermittent Fasting Affects Your Body

Intermittent fasting gained its popularity for its simplicity. You just have to follow a schedule on when you can eat and when you cannot. What's great about this simplicity is that it works.

Furthermore, the effects of intermittent fasting goes beyond weight loss. It also has positive effects to the hormones and cells that play a role in your overall and long-term health.

Here are some of the hormones, organs, and cells that intermittent fasting affects that, in turn, contribute to your overall health.

Decreased insulin levels and resistance

Insulin is a hormone produced by the pancreas. It is released when your blood sugar rises. Once released, it triggers the cells to absorb blood sugar. The cells would then use them for energy or, in the case of fat cells, store them for later use.

Insulin is a crucial hormone in the body's moderation of its blood sugar levels. It prompts the liver if there is too much of it to prevent complications arising from hyperglycemia like cardiovascular disease, and damage on the nerves and kidneys.

Unfortunately, we often experience high blood sugar because of the carbohydrate-rich nature of today's diet. This causes frequent spikes in insulin levels that eventually lead to the body developing insulin resistance. This increased resistance results to the body requiring higher levels of insulin to regulate its' blood sugar levels.

This high insulin resistance would eventually manifest in a variety of symptoms such as fatigue, increased belly fat, elevated fasting blood sugar, high blood pressure, and carbohydrate cravings. For women, it could even cause acquired polycystic ovarian syndrome and hair loss.

This body's abnormal resistance to the hormone can be broken through fasting. This is due to the practice of increasing the production of proteins that improve insulin sensitivity.

This was observed from a group of Muslims fasting during the season of Ramadan. The good news is that you do not need to follow their practice of fasting from dawn to sunset for 30 days. You can replicate the same results through the easier and shorter fasting regimen that intermittent fasting can provide.

Increased human growth hormone production

Human growth hormone plays a role in inducing growth during childhood, and reaches its peak production during one's teenage years. This slowly declines with age, but it still plays a role in the body's tissue repair, energy, metabolism, brain function and muscle growth. It is produced by your pituitary gland, the pea-sized gland found at the lower part of your brain.

The body increases the production of growth hormone during fasted states while asleep or awake. This increase is caused by the decline in the released insulin six hours after eating a meal. Growth hormone levels start to increase after 6 more hours and reach the highest amounts around 18 to 20 hours into the fast. This increase can go up to as much as 2000% as one's average levels and can last for up to 48 hours.

Improved cellular repair

Fasting is among the ways to trigger autophagy in the body. Autophagy is the self-cleaning process done by cells to break down and recycle its damaged organelles and molecules. Although it is a constant process, autophagy increases dramatically when the body's insulin level drops during a fasted state.

The increased cell repair during a fasted state is believed to be the cause of the increased longevity among humans and other organisms that consume a low caloric diet. It arises from how stem cells can regain their regenerative ability through cellular repair. This results to stem cells being able to recover the damage to tissue at a rate that was only possible at a younger age.

Improved resistance from oxidative damage

Free radicals occur naturally in the body because of the various metabolic processes in it or the exposure from external sources. The antioxidants produced by your body and obtained from your diet neutralize these to prevent damage to the molecules that make up your cells.

Unfortunately, there will be cases wherein the body has an excess amount of free radicals. This could even be the norm for those who have a poor diet or lifestyle that both contribute to low levels of antioxidants. In such cases, the cells suffer from chronic oxidative stress that leads to damage to their structures. If left unchecked, it could trigger conditions such as heart disease, diabetes, chronic inflammation, neurodegenerative diseases, and cancer.

Fasting can address this and even improve the body's resistance to oxidative damage. This is thanks to the increased production of the gene SIRT3. This gene helps prevent the production of free radicals and improve the processes that reverse the damage done on the cells and its organelles.

Improved heart health

The increased insulin levels brought about by chronically high blood sugar and insulin resistance increases the risk for developing cardiovascular disease. This risk further increases when combined with the complications brought about by the same conditions – obesity and high cholesterol levels.

As previously mentioned, a fasted state will dramatically decrease one's insulin levels. If done consistently through an intermittent fasting schedule, it can eventually bring one's insulin sensitivity back to normal levels. With the improved insulin sensitivity, one can reach a healthier weight, lower their body fat composition, and reduce their blood cholesterol levels. Since these markers have improved, there is a lower chance for heart disease as well.

Better brain function

The improved moderation of blood sugar levels, and reduced oxidative stress and inflammation brought about by intermittent fasting can also improve your brain function. This is due to the neurons switching from cell growth and reproduction to resource conservation and stress resistance. When this happens, the cells remove damaged molecules and dysfunctional organelles. This results to cells with better quality. These neurons would then reproduce when they shift back to growing and reproducing once you eat after fasting.

Also, fasting increases the levels of a hormone known as brain-derived neurotrophic factor (BDNF). This hormone is a critical component in the brain for learning, memory storage and recall, and neuron generation. Also, it helps brain cells to be resistant to stress caused by free radicals, fatigue, and your environment.

Possible prevention of chronic diseases related to cell health

The wastes, damaged molecules, and dysfunctional organelles, especially the mitochondria, increase the risk for diseases such as cancer, Alzheimer's and Parkinson's. With fasting triggering autophagy, these unwanted elements in your cells are flushed out. This could possibly be the reason why fasting has been observed to provide nerves with protection from mechanisms that cause Alzheimer's disease. In addition, it has been observed that short-term fasting can improve the effects of cancer treatment while improving the patient's tolerance against chemotherapy.

Better gene expression

Gene expression is the process of converting instructions found in our DNA into a useable product. This is what gives our cells the capability to respond to the different changes that happen in our environment. The responses often result in the form of proteins that would then trigger functions within the cell. Examples of these functions include immune response to a bacterial infection, protective response to a detected disease, and hormonal response to changes inside or outside the body.

The numerous gene expressions that happen in our different cells can degrade due to inflammation, oxidative stress, aging, and toxins. This degradation can sometimes lead to the onset of age-related and chronic illnesses and symptoms.

Intermittent fasting has been found to induce changes in the gene expressions. These changes have been noticed to improve the malformed gene expressions that increase the risk for chronic illnesses like heart disease .

Less hunger and more satiety for certain individuals

Your body feels hunger and satiety due to the hormones released by your body. The one that makes you feel hungry is known as ghrelin while the hormone that makes you feel full is leptin. These hormones are produced from your stomach and fat cells when certain conditions are met.

Women experience an increase in the production of appetite suppressing hormones while going through a schedule of long-term fasting. However, this decrease is not observed among men with healthy body compositions. In fact, leptin decreases after undergoing a schedule of intermittent fasting.

Moreover, women are more likely to maintain their weight after returning to their regular eating schedule. This is attributed to the higher levels of the hormone suppressing the appetite that resulted from intermittent fasting.

Chapter 6: Intermittent Fasting for Women

Because it's so important to divide research and studies of IF between men and women, I wanted to make this book oriented towards only women's health and productivity with weight loss during times of intermittent fasting. That being said, there will be no more mention of men in this book. We'll focus on women and get straight to the point.

When you engage with IF as a woman, you will encounter struggles unique to your body. You may have to tweak your method, your timing, and your approach numerous times until you perfect your practice to what's the most healthy and productive for you. This chapter will go over some of the basics of your hormones, your body, and your mental health, all about what IF can do for the situation inside.

By the end of this chapter, you should be armed with information that will strengthen your IF practice and help you know how to succeed even when you come up against internal hardship. You should feel more confident in how to alter your eating pattern to kick-start your metabolism without losing any of the good things your body does for you. You should feel interested in beginning or planning your lifelong intermittent fast.

Hormones & Health: Weight Loss

When it comes to female hormones, reproductive health takes internal and unspoken precedence over the weight concerns of the conscious individual. This primacy of reproductive health stands out more so with females than it does with males, as we discovered in the last chapter through the 2013 rat studies and more. However, there have to be bigger biological reasons behind that increased sensitivity.

The cause seems to be kisspeptin, which is a molecule similar to a protein that helps neurons communicate with each other about hunger and energy and more. This molecule exists in both males and females, but females have far more kisspeptin than males do, making them even more sensitive to energetic changes in their internal balances.

Therefore, when females' bodies release hormones like leptin, ghrelin, and insulin (that make them feel hungry or full), their brains and internal systems are already that much more inclined to "hear" those feelings and respond to reestablish balance. Women are therefore more likely to struggle with weight loss and general health problems related to increased sensitivity. Despite your body's natural processes, however, you can **absolutely** learn how to make intermittent fasting work for you and still maintain your ideal weight, health, and productivity.

IF & the Female Body

Since intermittent fasting is not so much a diet as it is an altered pattern in eating times and frequency, its relationship with the female body is not the same as the standard diet's relationship would be. In fact, it's not necessarily supportive for females to practice a strict diet while intermittent fasting, for the combination of the two, can work serious havoc on the female body itself.

To counteract any curious side-effects of IF on your physical and mental states, you can try and make sure to eat as nutritious a selection of food as you can, whenever possible. Furthermore, you can try not to **over**exert yourself through exercise, especially since you're altering your food and nutrition intake significantly. Also, you can ensure that you're not forcing yourself to engage in IF if you're ill, suffering from an infection, or struggling with a chronic disorder of some kind. Finally, if your body is already exhausted from work or struggles with anxiety (or otherwise), you might not want to put yourself through additional stress with a new pattern of eating.

The most important thing to do as you begin to engage with intermittent fasting as a female-bodied person is to make sure you're as connected to (and introspective of) your body as you can be, as often as you're able to be. The more you know your body and its tendencies (i.e. the frequency of your period, your tendencies with metabolism, your fat storage areas, your most common moods, your emotional crutches, etc.), the more successful your experiences with intermittent fasting can be.

Physical Effects of IF for Women

While the general effects of intermittent fasting include increased energy overall, clearer cognition and memory, improved immunity, slowed aging process, better heart health, increased insulin sensitivity, and more, are some of the physical effects for women deserve a little more detail in specific. For women, those specific details include:

lowered blood pressure in about two months or less, lowered cholesterol by ¼ the original toxic amount, better blood sugar control, decreased likelihood for type 2 diabetes, lowered chances of cancer, potential for increased muscle mass (with the ability to preserve it longer!), increased lifespan by up to 50 years, and increased awareness of internal bodily processes in general.

After a few months of intermittent fasting practice, you're sure to feel that your senses are somewhat heightened compared to how they were before, that your body works better and smoother than ever, that your weight melts off like wax from a candle, and that your mind and cognition are clearer than ever before.

Some physical effects function almost like warning signs for the woman practicing IF, too. If you experience poorer skin conditions, complete insomnia, loss of hair, excessive or shocking decrease in muscle mass, loss of period entirely, heart arrhythmia, or increased inflammations (whether internally or externally), you'll definitely want to consider altering your process, stopping the IF for a while, or visiting a nearby doctor for advice.

Using IF to Help with Periods, Fertility, and Metabolism

If you struggle monthly through painful periods; if you know you don't want to have children and you're not concerned about future fertility; or if you want to kick-start your metabolism to help yourself lose weight, all you have to do is start intermittently fasting without any concern whatsoever. If you're looking for hard and fast changes for your harsh menses, your fertility, or your weight issues, work your way up to fasting a few days a week, and you're sure to see the side-effects you seek played out within a month or two.

If you're interested in getting help with painful periods without substantial effects on your future fertility, simply make sure to get enough fat in your diet and supplemental estrogen (which you can find over the counter in a variety of forms). By making sure to consume enough healthy fat and by not restricting your caloric intake too much, you can use intermittent fasting to ease difficult menses without it having too much effect on your metabolism at the moment, and with it having hardly any effect on your fertility later on.

If you want the metabolism boost without effect on your periods or fertility, here's what you can do. Make sure you're eating enough healthy fats, but restrict caloric intake slightly, not too much though, mind you! You don't want to hurt those hunger hormones or inhibit your ability to ovulate and have a healthy period!

For these reasons, you should make sure **not** to intentionally or fastidiously "diet" while you're intermittently fasting but seeing as how you **do** want to lose weight and kick-start that metabolism, you can do **something** to help your body remember not to hang onto too much excess! That "**something**" that works so well is two-part: (1) once you define your method, keep to its timing strictly and; (2) when you have your meals, don't overindulge, binge, or gorge yourself; allow your caloric intake to be limited, but only slightly, as you work with IF.

Chapter 7: What is the difference between Burning Fat and Weight Loss

One of the biggest misconceptions created by the weight loss industry is that fat burning and losing weight is the same thing. Truth can't be farther from that. You can be losing weight without burning even a gram of fat in your body, and that is not going to help you at all. On the other hand, you may be burning a lot of fat. However, your weight may not go down at all.

Weight loss and fat burn are two different things. When you are burning fat and building muscles, your weight may not go down at all. On the contrary, you may even notice a slight increase in your weight while there would be a considerable reduction in your waistline and fat deposits at your hips and thighs. In that case, you would be making great progress as you would be losing dangerous visceral fat in your body, but building muscles at the same time. It means you would be getting healthier and stronger.

The muscles are compact but weigh more, while the fat is voluminous but weighs less. Therefore, even if you lose fat, you can gain weight. In that case, a slight increase in your weight wouldn't be a problem as your overall health would improve considerably, and you would lose the dangerous visceral fat at the same time.

Intermittent fasting has the ability to bring this positive change into your body. It creates the right conditions in your body, which allow the burning of fat and building of muscles. You will be able to burn your body fat faster than any other process as the main objective of the process to initiate fat burning

Chapter 8: What is Autophagy?

Autophagy is the relatively newfound ability that cells have, enabling them to recycle their parts that aren't working, to clear up the muck, to get rid of what's unhelpful, and to throw out their trash essentially. And what Autophagy gets rid of also are technically pathogenic microbes such as mold, fungus, bacteria, the virus that may be sitting in the cell that causes potential disorders, conditions, or diseases when they're allowed to stay in the cell.

Autophagy is an amazing physiological process, for its effects go as far as healing the brain, increasing and furthering anti-aging capacities, and significantly boosting immunity. It really goes to show that intermittent fasting enacts wide-spread healing on the body, rather than just helping it lose weight or look younger.

Protein Cycling is also related to Autophagy in that it helps your body and your cells work to recycle what isn't working through phases of protein consumption. Essentially, Protein Cycling is a process you can engage in to increase the anti-aging capacity of your intermittent fasting practice. What you do is alternate between times where you eat a lot of protein and times where you hardly eat any. When you're eating a lot of protein, you'll have high insulin levels and low glucagon (a hormone that works alongside yet opposite insulin to keep glucose levels in the blood at balance). But when you switch to low protein levels, your insulin levels will lower and glucagon levels will spike, meaning that (scientifically and physiologically) Autophagy is active and working in the body.

Autophagy, Protein Cycling, and Women's Health

When women decide to take command of their health, incredible things can happen. Whether you're older or younger, Autophagy as a process in the body is one of those incredible things, and it happens without you even thinking about it. However, you can also make choices that increase the occurrence of Autophagy, which only makes those incredible things in your body (your potential for self-guided healing, etc.) have a more profound effect.

For menopausal women, in particular, Autophagy creates a turnover of cells that helps the transition from young to mature. It helps in keeping these women's skin young, their limbs lose, their moods bright, and their transitions smooth overall. For women of all other ages, Autophagy gets rid of the gunk that keeps holding you back. It helps you move into new growth as well as the next stage of life with confidence. For women's health overall, Autophagy is utterly vital, and Protein Cycling only aids its occurrence and proper function.

How IF Affects People (concerning to Autophagy)

When paired with Protein Cycling, intermittent fasting can enact substantial and long-lasting healing for the body and the individual as a whole. Intermittent fasting, of course, effects people like a jolt to their systems, helping things be more productive and efficient. Also, IF causes Autophagy in the body, encouraging the cells to get rid of their "trash" and be healthier overall. When paired with Protein Cycling, though, intermittent fasting becomes almost like a real-world video game "cheat," but for weight loss, mental prowess, anti-aging abilities, and general well-being.

With Autophagy happening in the body, which only happens during low protein-intake or fasting states, your organs, your skin, your cells, your brain, your limbs, and more get a jolt of self-cleansing potential, and that possibility is incredible. You can take full advantage of that opportunity in yourself by engaging in conscious fasting in whatever intermittent plan works best for you.

As always, you may have to work through several methods to find the right one. But as long as you're Protein Cycling (an action inherent to intermittent fasting) in any regard, you'll ignite Autophagy and by doing so, you'll unintentionally save your own life again and again. What more could you ask for?

Chapter 9: Types of Intermittent Fasting

Crescendo Method

The crescendo method of intermittent fasting is the one voted most productive for female-bodied practitioners. This method is well-known for its gentle approach to fasting, its caution, and awareness of hormonal balance, its ability to help you lose weight, and its gradual introduction (which works especially well for women with inconsistent work or life schedules).

Through the crescendo method, the individual will fast 12 to 16 hours at a time for two or three days a week that is not consecutive days. For instance, she might fast Sunday, normally eat Monday and Tuesday, fast Wednesday, normally eat Thursday, fast Friday, eat normally on Saturday, and repeat the pattern the next Sunday. During fast days, light cardio exercises or yoga can be practiced, but no intense workouts are allowed, due to the long hours involved in the fast. As needed, drink lots of water (with salt added if/when you get dizzy!) and coffee if you desire any energy boosts.

After two successful weeks of this pattern of fasting, additional days can be added, or the timing can be tweaked based on what's working and what isn't. Intermittent Fasting is a way to lose weight that involves a structured program of when you should eat and when you should not eat. You will be able to create your own plan that will suit your needs, especially if you can go through with it quickly for a whole day! Quick means spending twelve full hours empty before a meal.This method amps up the power after the initial detoxification period, based on the abilities and reach of the individual. It builds in effect, but the impact remains the same such as increased health and decreased weight while respecting hormones and the potential for hefty mood swings.

16/8 method

This is the most popular approach to intermittent fasting. It involves a fasting phase of 16 hours and an eating phase of 8 hours within a single day. This means, if you start your eating phase at 11 in the morning, you will stop eating and start fasting at 7 in the evening.

The said fasting phase would then end at 11AM on the next day.

You are free to set the time for your eating and fasting phase. This makes it easy for you to tailor your own intermittent fasting plan to a schedule that would work best for your lifestyle.

The lean gains method falls under this approach. It has the same 16 hours of fasting and 8 hours of eating. However, it was designed for those with a highly active lifestyle such as athletes, weight trainers, and fitness enthusiasts.

The lean gains method places an importance on caloric intake for better fat loss and, at the same time, muscle gain. It also has recommendations on which macronutrient and how much caloric intake work best for the first meal after fasting, pre-workout meals, or rest day meals.

Eat-stop-eat method

The key to this method is that there should be a meal at least once every day. This means that you should have had eaten a meal before starting a 24-hour fasting phase that starts, for example, at 9 in the morning.

Like the 16/8 method, you can set the start of your fasting phase whenever you want. But, most people following this method choose to set their fasting period from 6PM until 6PM of the next day. This way they do not sleep hungry, which would often be the case for those just starting intermittent fasting.

20:4 Method

Stepping things up a notch from the 14:10 and 16:8 methods, the 20:4 method is a tough one to master, for it is rather unforgiving. People talk about this method of intermittent fasting as intense and highly restrictive, but they also say that the effects of living this method are almost unparalleled with all other tactics.

For the 20:4 method, you'll fast for 20 hours each day and squeeze all your meals, all your eating, and all your snacking into 4 hours. People who attempt 20:4 normally have two smaller meals or just one large meal and a few snacks during their 4-hour window to eat, and it really is up to the individual which four hours of the day they devote to eating.

The trick for this method is to make sure you're not over-eating or bingeing during those 4-hour windows to eat. It is all-too-easy to get hungry during the 20-hour fast and have that feeling then propel you into intense and unrealistic hunger or meal sizes after the fast period is over. Be careful if you try this method. If you're new to intermittent fasting, work your way up to this one gradually, and if you're working your way up already, only make the shift to 20:4 when you know you're ready. It would surely disappoint if all your progress with intermittent fasting got hijacked by one poorly thought-out goal with 20:4 method.

The Warrior Diet

The Warrior Diet is called such due to the belief that it was how ancient Paleolithic humans ate at the time. This diet involves a fasting phase of little to no food during the day and an eating phase of consuming as much food as desired.

The fasting phase starts from the moment of waking up during the day. It would last for 20 hours wherein it is encouraged to consume dairy products, raw fruits and vegetables, eggs, and non-caloric beverages in small amounts.

Once the 20-hour fasting phase ends, you are free to "feast" as much as you desire. This eating phase is said to be patterned after how the Spartan and Roman warriors would feast at night after a hard day's work.

As the name implies, the Warrior Diet goes beyond the simple eating and fasting schedule of the other intermittent fasting methods. It involves an actual diet that aims to improve the body's utilization of fat for its metabolism.

Also, it is encouraged for the one following it to take daily multivitamins, probiotics, and amino acids. It is also said to work best while doing a workout plan for increasing strength and speed to lose as much fat as possible during the diet's duration.

Lean-Gains Method (14:10)

The lean-gains method has several different incarnations on the web, but its fame comes from the fact that it helps shed fat while building it into muscle almost immediately. Through the lean-gains method, you'll find yourself able to shift all that fat to be muscle through a rigorous practice of fasting, eating right, and exercising.

Through this method, you fast anywhere from 14 to 16 hours and then spend the remaining 10 or 8 hours each day engaged in eating and exercise. This method, as opposed to the crescendo, features daily fasting and eating, rather than alternated days of eating versus not. Therefore, you don't have to be quite so cautious about extending the physical effort to exercise on the days you are fasting because those days when you're fasting are literally every day!

For the lean-gains method, start fasting only 14 hours and work it up to 16 if you feel comfortable with it, but never forget to drink enough water and be careful about expending too much energy on exercise! Remember that you want to **grow** in health and potential through intermittent fasting. You'll certainly not want to lose any of that growth by forcing the process along.

One Meal a Day (OMAD)

The One Meal a Day method utilizes a 23-hour fasting phase and a 1-hour eating phase. This would be just enough for you to have a single meal each day. It is a more advanced method compared to the Warrior Diet. You would also be more likely eating less calories in it since you only have an hour to eat.

5:2 method

The 5:2 method derives its name from the five days of normal eating and the two days of fasting involved for a single week. Unlike the other methods, this method does not involve a complete restriction from food during the fasting phases. Instead, the fasting phases come in the form of restricting food intake to 25 percent of a person's daily calorie intake.

These calorie-restricted days can be scheduled whichever day that you want. However, there should always be at least a single day of normal eating between the fasting days.

There is no restriction on one's food choices during the fasting days. There is also no limit on the number of meals in it as long as the total calories does not exceed the limit. Like the modified approach to alternate day fasting, you can spread out the calories for the day to two to three meals.

The common practice for this method is to schedule the fasted days during the weekdays. In this way, they would not be missing out on social events where food is likely involved.

Alternate day fasting (ADF)

The alternate day fasting, or ADF, involves a full day of fasting every other day. This method could be done by a fast that starts the moment you wake up until the time you wake up the next day, or by starting to fast in the evening and ending it after 24 hours. Unlike the eat stop eat method, you will be fasting every other day.

With this method, you are encouraged to drink as much calorie-free beverage that you can. This would include water, and unsweetened tea and coffee. Some would argue that the tea and coffee should have no dairy as well since these contain sugars that your body converts to calories.

You can modify this method so it does not involve a complete restriction from food during the fasting phase. Instead, you can limit your total caloric limit to 25 to 30 percent of your daily calories spread out to two to three meals within the day. In this way, you can stave off the feeling of hunger but still remain on a fasted state. Unlike the two day low calorie fasts of the 5:2 method, you will eat a low amount of calories on alternating days of the week.

12:12 Method

As another of the easier methods of intermittent fasting, 12:12 method is well-suited to beginning practitioners. Many people actually live out 12:12 method without any forethought simply because of their sleeping and eating schedule but turning 12:12 into a conscious practice can have just as many positive effects on your life as the more drastic 20:4 method claims.

For this method, in particular, you fast for 12 hours and then enter a 12-hour eating window. It's not difficult whatsoever to get three small meals and several snacks, or two big meals and a snack into your day with this method. With 12:12, the standard meal timing works just fine. For instance, many of us already stop eating at 8 or 9 o'clock at night and then wait until 8 or 9 o'clock the next morning for breakfast. With this 12-hour gap between meals, these people are unintentionally already professionals at 12:12 method.

Ultimately, this method is a great one to start from, for a lot of variation can be built into this scheduling when you're ready to make things more interesting. Easily and without much effort, 12:12 can become 14:10 or even 16:8, and in seemingly no time, you can find yourself trying alternate-day or crescendo methods, too. Start with what's normal for you, and this method might be exactly that!

Spontaneous Skipping Method

As the purposefully least-organized method of the bunch, spontaneous skipping method leaves most of the definition and planning to the individual. There's no easy division of time between fasting and feeding. There's no delineating of how much time needs to be spent on what. In fact, there are no standards for this plan whatsoever. The individual determines all this planning for him or herself.

In this case, all you need to do is skip one or two meals each day. That's all you need to do. Skip breakfast and your second snack one day, skip lunch and dinner the next (in favor of a bedtime snack), and then skip breakfast again the day after. Skip meals based on what's convenient for you, too!

If you're someone who has trouble defining a daily schedule, if you're someone who balks at routine, or if you're someone who works increasingly varying shifts at work; this intermittent fasting method is probably perfect for you. Try this one out to start or try it after you've realized some of the more "structured" methods don't work, based on your lifestyle. Regardless of how you do it, just try it! Even if you're not fully working at intermittent fasting quite yet, dip your toes in the water! Skip a meal here and then, and I promise, your body will thank you for it.

Chapter 10: Tips and Tricks to reach your best shape

Intermittent fasting has become more popular as the days go by. A lot of people want to give it a try. Here are a few tips and tricks that will help you reach your perfect shape during your intermittent fasting:

Keep short, fasting periods. There are different types of intermittent fasting, and you have to decide which one you will follow through. You choose one that you can easily incorporate in your lifestyle without much hustle. Doctors and nutritionists advise using shorter fasting periods, between 8 to 24 hours. The best option, according to several consultants, is 12 hours. A 12-hour fasting window is adequate to ensure you get the benefits of intermittent fasting without pushing your body to the limit. Fasting for long periods can have adverse effects on your body. For example, you feel dehydrated, your mood is affected, and you become irritable, inability to remain focused, low energy, among many others. If you are beginning your intermittent fasting journey, it is best to keep the fasting to a restricted timeframe.

Eat little amount on days you are fasting. Fasting generally is skipping meals or eating very little for that period. A good number of fasting types require you to abstain from food altogether. However, there are intermittent fasting types that allow you to eat a small portion of your regular calories during your fast days. For example, the 5: 2 type will enable you to take 25% of your regular calorie intake during the two days you decide to fast. Fasting is easier when you are restricting your calories, instead of abstaining from food altogether. It reduces the adverse side effects of not eating, and it is an easier way to maintain your intermittent fasting lifestyle.

Keep your body hydrated. By fasting, you already deny your body 20% of its source of hydration. To avoid being completely dehydrated, you have to drink plenty of water during the days you are fasting. Dehydration can cause you to feel tired, have headaches, and feel light-headed. It is recommended to drink about eight glasses of water a day to be adequately hydrated, though it also depends on the person in question. Listen to your body cues, like thirst, to know when to drink more water. Please note that drinking water is not only crucial during fasting days, but also important every other day. Keeping your body hydrated is an everyday task.

Walk or meditate. Avoiding food on days, you should fast, can be quite challenging, especially if you are still new to intermittent fasting. It is always good to keep yourself preoccupied. Take a walk around your home or wherever you are or meditate. These activities are not strenuous that they will use a lot of energy. They will help keep your mind off the topic of food and make your journey easier. Any other activity that can calm and engage your mind is also welcome, such as reading a book, taking a bath, or even sleeping.

Do not feast on the non-fast days. We are human, and since we are accustomed to eating now and then, we can be tempted to overindulge after fasting. We may want to make up for the fasting by eating more than we usually do, which is not advisable. Consuming more than usual may hinder you from moving forward. If you are trying to lose weight, taking more calories on non-fasting days will decrease the calorie deficit. You may end up gaining more weight because of the excessive calories you consume. Ending your fasting by consuming a lot of food will likely leave you feeling tired and bloated. It also slows down the positive effect of fasting. It is best to eat as you usually would after fasting, to stay on track.

If you feel sick, stop fasting. Fasting can make you feel hungry or tired, but you should not feel sick. If you are new to fasting, and even if you are not, try to limit your fasting period to 12 hours. Do not exceed 24 hours if you feel like 12 hours will not be sufficient for you. Always keep a snack near you just in case you feel faint. The moment you feel sick, stop fasting. The main aim of fasting is to improve your health, not make you ill. Signs that you should stop fasting and consult a doctor include feeling extreme discomfort and feeling too weak that normal daily tasks are challenging to perform. Your health is the priority; don't push yourself to the extent that you become too ill to function. Eat plenty of protein. One of the main goals of intermittent fasting is losing weight. However, since fasting includes restriction your calories, you may lose your muscle mass as well as the fats. Eating protein during intermittent fasting will help you retain your muscle mass while still losing weight. Also, taking little amounts of protein during fasting can help you feel full longer and keep your appetite at bay. Eating protein is an excellent way to reduce some of the side effects of fasting.

Eat whole foods when you are not fasting. One of the main goals of fasting is to improve the health of a person. You do this by maintaining a healthy and well-balanced diet during days you are not fasting. Healthy diets and consist of whole foods are beneficial to the body. They have several health benefits, which include the reduction in the risk of getting heart diseases, cancer, and other health-related illnesses. Your diet should contain whole foods such as legumes, fruits, vegetables, eggs, fish, and meat.

Take supplements. Fasting can cause someone to miss out on essential nutrients essential to the body. If losing weight is one of your objectives, you are likely not to get enough vitamin B12, calcium, and iron. Consider taking supplements to reduce the risk of deficiencies in the body.

Mild exercises. Some people can exercise while they fast and not be bothered by it. If you are new to fasting, keep exercising to a minimum to see how your body takes it. Do mild exercises like walking or stretching. Do not push yourself over the limit before your body gets the chance to be accustomed to fasting. Listen to what your body tells you and stop any exercising if you struggle too much.

Begin fasting after dinner. Whether you are fasting weekly or daily, one of the best pieces of advice you will receive is to begin your fast after you eat your dinner. This usually makes fasting easier because you spend a good portion of the time asleep. It helps keep your hunger in check, and time moves faster. It is especially helpful if you are beginning intermittent fasting. Your body will be trying to get used to not eating, and sleeping for most of the fasting period will make it a little easier.

Eating satiating meals. One of the main problems with fasting is feeling unsatisfied and hungry nearly all the time. You are continually craving food, or you feel like you need to eat more to feel at least satisfied. You dread the thought of having to repeat eating the same foods and feeling the same way nearly every day. Here comes in satiating meals. These are meals that keep you full for more extended periods and the feeling of hunger or wanting to eat. The good thing about intermittent fasting, unlike other diets, is the freedom to eat foods that you can enjoy and that offer satisfactions in the long run, provided they are healthy. Satiating meals include soups, oatmeal, bananas, eggs, yogurt, and potatoes. Satiating meals should not cause you to deviate from your healthy diets. They should be part of your fat loss diet, meaning they need to be healthy and low in calories and carbs. Keep your appetite at bay. Appetite makes you feel hungry. Therefore, keeping it bay will help you manage to fast easily. You can reduce your appetite by drinking drinks that have no calories, such as water, green tea, black coffee, and sparkling water.

Give yourself time. To achieve your set goals for intermittent fasting, you have to start somewhere. You cannot start running before you walk. Your body needs time to adjust to the changed schedule. Let it adjust to not eating for more extended periods than it is used to.

Slowly get into the program you made for yourself, especially if it is your first time. You will find the beginning challenging, and you might backslide one, two, or a few times. It is only natural. Do not give up, though. Persevere through it and stick to your routine. It is the only way to reach your end goals and benefit from the journey. Patience is vital here.

Get into the right mindset. Intermittent fasting is not a temporary option for when every other option fails. It is a long process on its own, which will require a lot of persistence. It is essential to know that as much as it has its benefits, intermittent fasting relies on how consistent you are and you achieving your calorie goals. You need to have the right mindset for it to work. Three basic steps of getting into the correct mindset are: having realistic expectations from which you set your goals; be consistent and focus on achieving your set goal; and have patience, knowing that good things take time.

Enjoy yourself. Intermittent fasting gives you a lot of nutritional freedom that allows you to enjoy yourself whenever you want. It works on restricting your calories; therefore, if say you have a function in the evening, you are free to skip breakfast and enjoy yourself in the evening. You being on a diet don't mean that you can't take time to enjoy other meals with others. You may have to limit your intake for another time, but you are still able to indulge sometimes.

Chapter 11: Keep a Healthy lifestyle

When following intermittent fasting, you have to keep in mind that even though you are eating very healthy and that you are taking care of your body having a good workout routine is recommended. Once you figured out what kind of intermittent fasting plan you're going to be following, make sure that you get a workout plan that will help you to put on muscle or lose body fat whichever your goal is.

One of the great things about intermittent fasting is that you can lose weight or gain muscle while following this method, which is why many people consider intermittent fasting one of the best eating plans to follow, for overall health and wellness. By now, you know everything about intermittent fasting and how you should be following, especially for women as it is different than men when it comes to intermittent fasting. To understand how to stay healthy when intermittent fasting, there are some things you need to take care of before you start intermittent fasting. The first one would be to make sure that you have a proper workout plan based on your goals, there are many workout plans which you can find online that will help you to come up with a workout plan based on your goals. Keep in mind that you will have to work hard to come up with a workout plan if you're not an expert. If you can afford to get a personal trainer, then get one, as it will help you create a great workout plan for your needs. However, finding a workout plan online isn't so hard, and you can do so by looking up online for a bit.

Another thing you need to make sure when intermittent fasting is that you need to take care of your diet, even though you are allowed to eat whatever you want when intermittent fasting you need to make sure that your diet is a lot healthier if your goal is to lose weight. Don't get me wrong, and you will still lose weight when following intermittent fasting; however, making sure that you are eating very healthy, then you will see better results overall. Finally, you need to make sure that you're taking care of yourself internally. Make sure they are getting enough micronutrients throughout the day to support your health.

Another thing to keep in mind would be that you will lose fat most of the time when fasting instead of the weight. Keep in mind, when fasting, you will gain muscle and lose fat, which might not make you lose weight but instead fat. As always do body measurements instead of bodyweight check overall?

There are many ways to do that, but one of the best ways to go about it would be to take multivitamins during your eating window. Keep in mind that if you take multivitamins when you are fasting will break the fast, so make sure that you're not taking multivitamins during your fast but in fact after you're fast. Finally, make sure that you do everything in conjunction if your goal is to see amazing results. There is no better way to see results, and if you combine all three aspects, then you will be in a much better position to truly reap the benefits out of it. With that being said, we conclude this book, thank you so much for sticking thru.

Chapter 12: Which diet to choose?

Because you'll likely want to keep your reproductive and menstrual systems working to their best capacities while you engage in intermittent fasting, you'll have to make sure your dietary choices reflect the health you want to see. You won't really want to "diet" all that much, as mentioned above, but you can make certain healthful changes that allow your body to function at its highest capacity **while** it adjusts to intermittent fasting, sheds that excess weight, and reaches a new and purer energy level than you've ever experienced before.

In this chapter, you will be introduced to concepts and details that will help you eat and drink the things that are best suited to your overall growth and success with intermittent fasting. You'll be shown the pros and cons of the intermittent fasting lifestyle, and you'll be taught tips on how to manage hunger and generally achieve your IF goals.

By the end of this section, you should know the best and worst that intermittent fasting has to offer, and you should feel confident that the foods you'll seek during your break from fast will be as health-conscious and supportive as possible, based on the information you've gained. Finally, you should also feel prepared to deal with those "worsts" that IF has to offer through the tips at the end of the chapter. If you're not ready to try intermittent fasting by the end of this section, I'll be incredibly surprised.

Pros & Cons of IF as a Dietary/Lifestyle Choice

On the most basic level (without being too redundant), the pros of switching to intermittent fasting (whether as a lifestyle choice or as more of a simple two-month fasting experiment) include:

Increased health overall

through weight loss, lowered insulin & blood sugar levels, heart health, better muscle mass preservation, increased neuroplasticity, potential for cancer healing, lower blood pressure & cholesterol, healthier hormone production, longer life, re-started/re-inspired nutrient absorption, reduced inflammation

Increased energy, improved mental processing and better access to memory

Increased overall sense of well-being

both mentally and as a side-effect of having the body type you want through weight loss

Eased & regulated menstruation

including lessened period cramps and potential for lessened fertility

The ability to retain your current diet and caloric intake

The overall simplicity and ease of starting and maintaining your IF approach, and the versatility and flexibility of IF as a practice

On the flip-side, the cons associated with intermittent fasting   (as both a lifestyle and momentary dietary choice) include:

Potential for increased headaches

These are often caused by dehydration and salt withdrawal from eating less than normal.

Increase your water intake & mix in a quarter-teaspoon of salt with each water glass, and you'll feel right as rain in no time.

Potential for constipation

Just increase your fiber intake to help with this issue!

Potential for dizziness when in a fasting period

Look to the final section of this chapter for help in this case.

 Potential for muscle cramps

Take supplemental magnesium or sit for a while in an Epsom salt bath to cure these "growing" pains.

Potential for worst-case-scenario side-effects

This potential is only a concern if IF is not practiced the right way for you and your body.

potential side-effects include: irregular or ceased menses, hair loss, dry skin/acne, slow healing to injuries, mood swings, super-slow metabolism, constant cold feelings, insomnia, etc.

Potential to binge when you do eat

Be conscious of your body and what it can handle!

Interference with social eating patterns

It might feel awkward not to eat with everyone else, or to have to explain yourself every time you don't.

Low energy or unproductivity during fast periods

This issue can be helped with practice and by eating the right types of foods when you do eat.

The fact that some of the lasting effects of IF are still largely unstudied or uncertain

such as: its effects on the heart, on fertility, on breastfeeding women, on stress, etc.

What Foods & Liquids Do

When you go about your first round of intermittent fasting, you'll need to know what to avoid and what to keep close at hand. The following portion of this chapter will reveal exactly what's safe, what to avoid, and what does what for you.

When it comes to foods, the best things to have around are:

All Legumes and Beans – good carbs can help lower body weight without planned calorie restriction

Anything high in protein – helpful in keeping your energy levels up in your efforts as a whole, even when you're in a period of fasting

Anything with the herbs cayenne pepper, psyllium, or dried/crushed dandelion – they'll contribute to weight loss without sacrificing calories or effort

Avocado – a high-, good-calorie fruit that has a lot of healthy fats

Berries – often high in antioxidants and vitamin C as well as flavonoids for weight loss

Cruciferous Vegetables – broccoli, cauliflower, brussel sprouts, and more are incredibly high in fiber, which you'll definitely want to keep constipation at bay with IF

Eggs – high in protein and great for building muscle during IF periods

Nuts & Grains – sources of healthy fats and essential fiber

Potatoes – when prepared in healthy ways, they satiate hunger well and help with weight loss

Wild-Caught Fish – high in healthy fats while providing protein and vitamin D for your brain

When it comes to liquids, some of it is pretty self-explanatory:

Water:

It's always good for you! It will help keep you hydrated, it will provide relief with headaches or lightheadedness or fatigue, and it clears out your system in the initial detox period.

Try adding a squeeze of lemon, some cucumber or strawberry slices, or a couple of sprigs of mint, lavender, or basil to give your water some flavor if you're not enthused with the taste of it plain.

If you need something other than water to drink, you can always seek out:

Probiotic drinks like kefir or kombucha

You can even look for probiotic foods such as sauerkraut, kimchi, miso, pickles, yogurt, tempeh, and more!

Probiotics work amazingly well at healing your gut especially in times of intense transition, as with the start of intermittent fasting.

Black coffee

Sweeteners and milk aren't productive for your fasting and weight loss goals.

Try black coffee whenever possible, in moderation.

Heated or chilled vegetable or bone broths

Teas of any kind

Apple cider vinegar shots

Instead, try water or other drinks with ACV mixed in.

Drinks to avoid would be:

Regular soda

Diet soda

Alcohol of any kind

High-sugar coconut and almond drinks

i.e. coconut water, coconut milk, almond milk, etc.

Go for the low-sugar or unsweetened milk alternative if it's available.

Anything with artificial sweetener

Artificial sweetener will shock your insulin levels into imbalance with your blood sugar later on.

Managing Hunger & Other Useful Tips

A few supportive tips to help troubleshoot, keep inspired and stay focused as you may happen to encounter the "cons" of intermittent fasting are as follows.

Generally, keep these pointers in mind: don't over-exercise and over-limit yourself with calorie intake or with food when you do breakfast. Take pictures of your progress to help keep the inspiration flowing, try not to binge when you breakfast and make sure to do your proper research or check with your doctor to be sure your plan for intermittent fasting is really the right one for you!

When it comes to managing hunger, the best thing to do is think of hunger like a wave passing over you.

Sometimes the build-up to that wave seems unbearable, but it will crest and crash eventually, passing completely over and through you. If you wait it out, keep yourself busy, and take a few sips of a drink instead. You'll find that these hunger pangs are bearable and not quite as overwhelming as they were at the start. By the end of the third day, you should have a significantly increased capacity to handle these feelings of hunger.

If you start feeling dizzy or lightheaded, one of two things is likely happening to you. You may be experiencing low blood volume, or you might be experiencing low blood **pressure** instead. Just drinking water, in this case, might not help you all that much; in fact, if you just drink water, you'll be diluting the number of electrolytes in your system even more, so try mixing a bit of sea salt in your water instead. Frequently, for those who don't experience dizziness or lightheadedness unless they're intermittently fasting, this addition of sea salt to water does the trick. However, some people were liable to feel dizzy or lightheaded before they ever tried IF. For those people (or for those for whom mixing salt into their water doesn't help), taking magnesium supplements can also work well, and if that still doesn't help, the issue could be something else entirely. Possible adrenal weakness, anemia, or low blood sugar would most likely be the cause in this case.

If your period gets lighter or starts to disappear, make sure you're getting enough fat in your diet when you fast! If you **had** been limiting calorie intake, stop doing that right now, and be sure not to binge (on the opposite extreme). Just eat what you would if you weren't IF or dieting at all. These slight adjustments should help resolve this issue. If not, seek advice from your doctor.

When you notice you've become moodier, there are a couple of things you can do to help and troubleshoot the issue. First things first, don't open yourself up to negative moods by keeping the information about your eating pattern shift to yourself and people you really trust. Some people will bombard you with questions, hate, or confusion when you tell them about your work with IF, and you should remember that you **don't** have to tell anyone who you think won't support you.

Second, you can make sure you're not still in the detox period of intermittent fasting! During the first few weeks, you'll be working through the detox period that brings up lots of literal stink and emotional issues to boot. Bear through the trial period and see if that moodiness lingers. If you're still frustratingly and unusually moody after week two is complete, you might just have low blood sugar. Work to counteract low blood sugar through the foods you choose to eat when you breakfast, and the issue should clear itself up in no time.

Finally, two pieces of advice are left, and they're some of the most important ones to internalize. First, **choose a plan that starts small and incorporates your life in its planning**! If you sleep for almost 12 hours each night anyway, the 16:8 method might be best for you. If you wake early without much sleep constantly, you might be better off doing alternate-day fasting. Go with what works for your schedule, and things will start off so much smoother than they would otherwise.

Second and lastly, **start with one month and be open; see what happens**! You're bound to get frustrated and moody after and during the first week but commit to withstand the awkwardness and at least get through the first two weeks to the beginning of week three. Stick with it and wait to see what this unintentional cleanse has in store for you.

Chapter 13: How to Start Intermittent Fasting?

Setting your expectations before committing to a fast is an excellent way of preparing both your body and mind for the lifestyle and dietary changes that are about to happen.

Before delving into the details of these expectations, you should be clear first about your personal objectives for the fast. Here are some common scenarios that have led people into fasting:

They want to lose weight, and gain a leaner body.

They have tried other popular diets before, and they felt dissatisfied with the process, or frustrated over the results.

They want to significantly improve the current condition of their body.

They want to be live a longer, healthier, and more productive life.

Fasting is a proven method of losing weight in a healthy manner, while increasing your energy levels. For many, it is a life-changing practice that have enabled them to achieve their other personal goals in life.

Committing to a fast requires determination and confidence that you can go through this without giving in to your old ways. You need plan and prepare for this because you might have to make drastic changes in your life.

For your guidance, here are the various things that you should expect for when starting a fast:

Grocery Shopping

Fasting would significantly change the way you shop for food. Aside from the frequency of your shopping days, some items from your current shopping list must be removed and replaced with healthier alternatives.

In general, you should stick to leaner types of proteins, such as certain types of fishes and egg whites. For fruits and vegetables, it is advisable to spend a bit more and buy organic produce.

Meal Restrictions

The exact meal schedule that you have to observe depends on the fasting method that you are following. However, all fasting methods would limit your calorie intake either by reducing the allowable number of calories, or by urging you to skip certain meals—if not all of them.

For example, a 5:2 diet imposes a 500-calorie limit among women, and 600-calorie limit among men. Both are significantly less than the recommended amount for average individuals.

Imbibing alcohol drinks during a fast is strongly discouraged as well. Even when you are on your "off days" from your fast, experts recommend only a moderate amount.

During a fast, you would also have to drink more water. If you prefer flavored beverages, then you should stick to herbal teas and black coffee with no sugar. Some health experts also allow drinking club soda during a fast.

Refer to chapter 4 of this book for more information about the meal restrictions of different fasting methods.

Physiological side-effects

Many of these side-effects can be considered as the disadvantages of fasting. However, with the right mindset, you would be able to power through them despite the challenges they might pose to your day-to-day life.

Hunger Pangs

Hunger is a natural reaction of the body when you begin abstaining from food. It is an unavoidable aspect of fasting, but it is not entirely a negative one. Studies show that hunger can actually increase your focus and improve your mental clarity.

Lightheadedness

It may take you some time to get used to being in a fasted state. During your adjustment period, you are likely going to experience lightheadedness and other uncomfortable bodily sensations. Those are perfectly normal, and they will go away once your body has fully adapted to the changes in your lifestyle.

Low Energy

Experiencing a drop in your energy levels is another short-term symptom that you should expect and prepare for during the initial stages of your fast.

Your body is used to getting a certain amount of calories per day. When you begin skipping your meals, your body would have to adjust and trigger other internal processes that could provide you the energy you need to perform normally.

According to experts, this period of low energy can last from one to two weeks. After that, you would be able to feel more energized even when you continue being in a fasted state.

Learning how to prepare yourself for this positive change in your life is important. It's best to switch to a low-carbohydrate, fatty diet for three weeks if anyone want to start intermittent fasting. It allows the body to use fat rather than sugar as an energy source. This involves the removal of all sugars, cereals (bread, cookies, pasta, rice), vegetables, and refined oils. This will minimize the most fasting side effects.

Start with a shorter pace of 16 hours, for instance, from dinner (8 pm) to lunch the next day (12 pm). You will usually eat between 12 and 20 pm and consume two or three meals. You can extend it quickly to 18, 20 hours once you feel comfortable with it.

For shorter fasts, you can do so continuously every day. You can do it 1-3 times a week for more prolonged fasts, such as 24-36 hours, alternating between fasting and regular eating days.

To better illustrate what you would go through during a fast, here is an overview of a typical intermittent and extended fasting period.

Your body will enter its fasting state at around 8 hours after your last meal. This is the average duration for a full digestion and complete absorption of nutrients from the food and beverages you have consumed prior to your fasting period.

It could vary, however, depending on the kind of meal you had—for instance, foods high in fiber need a longer digestive period compared to leafy vegetables.

During the initial fasting period, your body would still get most of its energy from your glucose stores, or also known as glycogen.

The glycogen stored in your liver would be depleted after an overnight fast.

Once completely your body has completely used up all the glucose stores in your body, it would begin sourcing energy from the fat stores within your body.

Take note, however, that the body is already converting fat into energy even before you have consumed all the glycogen in your body. Fasting only increases the rate of fat-burning, thus making it an effective means of losing excess weight.

There's no right fasting scheme. The essential thing is to choose one that works best for you. Some people get results with shorter fasts; others may require longer fasts. Some people make classic water-just fast; others make tea and coffee quickly, others a bone broth.

Regardless of what you do, keeping hydrated, and monitoring yourself is very important. You should stop immediately if you feel ill at any point. You might be hungry, but don't feel sick.

Knowing what to expect is critical in the long-term success of your fast. Realign your goals based on what you have learned from this chapter so that you can create a realistic and achievable fasting plan.

Chapter 14: Maintaining calories intake during fasting

The first and perhaps one of the most important parts of successfully eating the intermittent fasting diet without any serious side effects is maintaining a proper calorie count each day. Having a smaller eating window can make this more challenging, so it is important that you are eating properly during these windows. If you begin eating the intermittent fasting diet and do not receive enough calories, the impacts that you might experience could be quite negative. In addition to experiencing things like excessive hunger and headaches, you may also begin experiencing excessive weight loss. Weight loss on the intermittent fasting diet is a great side effect, but not if it is happening because you are quite literally starving. It is important that you discover what the healthy calorie intake is for your age and weight range. Then, make sure that you are incorporating that caloric intake into your eating window. This may mean that during your eating window you are eating fairly consistently in order to get in enough calories to remain healthy. Focus on eating calorie-dense foods that are high in nutrition, such as meats and vegetables, to get your intake up. This will ensure that you stay well-nourished and that you do not begin losing weight as a result of starvation.

When it comes to weight loss, it is the method, in recent years, that has been much more widely used. Fasting is not a new idea, and it's probably one of the oldest weight control methods, actually quite the contrary, but that's a whole different story.

Whether or not fasting is safe is the issue which the medical and nutritional experts have raised several times, more often than not, although both are beginning to be much more open-minded on this often controversial method of weight loss.

Fasting generally involves food, liquids, or both, and self-deprivation. Again, fasting can occur in various kinds, such as fasting of fruits, intermittent, only water, or vegetable juice, etc. In many cases, though, people will abstain entirely from food intake. Unfortunately, the answer to the question when it comes to achieving objectives of rapid weight loss... Fasting is secure, not as cut and dry as many would hope since the answer is yes and no!

Moderation is suitable for most things, and fasting is no different. If you fast for too long, the effects can be harmful and lead to diseases ranging from anorexia to liver failure. Still, fasting can provide many advantages regularly, including a colonic and clearer skin as well as a weight loss.

While it is 100% true that the numerous types of fasts help people to lose weight quickly, it can also be true that a lot of this weight is fluid and not fat, well at least at first and only if you were at full swing, when you don't eat water, or food, by the way!

The reasons why weight loss should not take fasting into account and why it ought to be! Confused?

1. Fasting is slowing down your metabolism. This means that the fat you try to lose begins to burn at a much slower rate, so you stop losing weight. This is true, but what is not emphasized is how long you need to be in a rapid state to slow down your metabolism.

Look at it this way, everyone else is on a diet or two, but what all foods do, is to reduce the daily calorie intake. What we find out with all diets is that they all reach a plateau of weight loss, most of them around the first two weeks. A plateau is when the weight loss process of the previous two weeks either slows down significantly or stops entirely.

The reason for this is that the metabolism of the body has adapted to the new low-calorie intake, and once done, it will stop the fat reserves from being burned. Fasting will have the same effect for a long time and will reach a plateau too. However, intermittent 24-hour fasting periods won't influence your metabolism but will STILL reduce your weekly calorific consumption.

2. Fasting is not recommended for people with health problems. If someone has a health disorder or is taking drugs, fasting should be avoided, since it can quickly worsen such problems or weaken the immune system of the person. A balanced person needs all the nutrients he can get, while every person who uses certain medications requires substantial digestive material to

safely ingest and even to help them work out their intended actions.

Most are right, but many medical conditions would greatly benefit from intermittent fasting, and there are alternative medications for most complaints that work without food. Remember, we're thinking about irregular fasting periods not approaching 24 hours, a quarter of which would be used to bed! I'm sure there are millions of Muslims and people from other religions that often take medicines safely and fast at the same time, for religious reasons. The safest option is to consult your doctor at all times.

Mostly, if fasting is safe depends entirely on the circumstances. If overlooked, it could pose a real danger to your wellbeing. Still, the path towards a healthy and natural weight loss is open if nutritional experts follow a sensible, easy guideline centered on scientifically proven ways.

First and foremost, hunger is unintentional abstinence from outside forces; it happens when food is scarce in times of and famine war. On the other hand, fasting is voluntary, deliberate, and monitored. Food is readily available, but we do not eat it for spiritual reasons, health reasons, or for other purposes.

Fasting does not have a regular duration. It can be done for a couple of hours to several days or months. Intermittent fasting is a mode of eating in which we cycle between fasting and regular food. In general, shorter 16-20-hour fasting is more frequent even daily. Longer fasts are done 2-3 times per week, usually 24-36 hours. As it happens, between dinner and breakfast, we all quickly spend about 12 hours each day.

Millions and millions of people have been fasting for thousands of years. Is it healthy? Is it healthy? No. No. Many studies have shown that it has enormous health benefits.

CONCLUSION

I'd like to thank you and congratulate you for transiting my lines from start to finish.

I hope this book was able to help you to discover the right fasting method for you.

The next step is to apply what you have learned from this book by creating a fasting plan that would work with your current lifestyle and help you achieve your personal fitness goals.

You should also go for a consultation with your physician as well in order to get their opinion about your plan to fast. Make sure that you would be able to fully commit to fasting once you have begun. Though the planning stage may take a long time, you should push through until you are completely certain about the details pertaining to this life-changing decision.

I wish you the best of luck!